D1552064

{WITHDRAWN}

WILLIAM F. MAAG LIBRARY
YOUNGSTOWN STATE UNIVERSITY

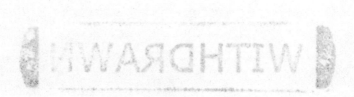

The Child's Eye

OXFORD MEDICAL PUBLICATIONS

The Child's Eye
Diagnosis of Ophthalmic
Disorders in Children

B. DHILLON
Consultant Ophthalmic Surgeon BMedSci., BMBS, FRCS (Glasg.) FRCOphth
Princess Alexandra Eye Pavilion, Edinburgh

and

G. T. MILLAR
Consultant Ophthalmic Surgeon MBChB, DRCOG, FRCS (Edin.) FRCOphth
Princess Alexandra Eye Pavilion, Edinburgh

Oxford   New York   Tokyo
OXFORD UNIVERSITY PRESS
1994

Oxford University Press, Walton Street, Oxford OX2 6DP

Oxford   New York   Toronto
Delhi   Bombay   Calcutta   Madras   Karachi
Kuala Lumpur   Singapore   Hong Kong   Tokyo
Nairobi   Dar es Salaam   Cape Town
Melbourne   Auckland   Madrid
and associated companies in
Berlin   Ibadan

Oxford is a trade mark of Oxford University Press

Published in the United States
by Oxford University Press Inc., New York

© *B. Dhillon and G. T. Millar, 1994*

All rights reserved. No part of this publication may be
reproduced, stored in a retrieval system, or transmitted, in any
form or by any means, without the prior permission in writing of Oxford
University Press. Within the UK, exceptions are allowed in respect of any
fair dealing for the purpose of research or private study, or criticism or
review, as permitted under the Copyright, Designs and Patents Act, 1988, or
in the case of reprographic reproduction in accordance with the terms of
the licences issued by the Copyright Licensing Agency. Enquiries concerning
reproduction outside these terms and in other countries should be sent to
the Rights Department, Oxford University Press, at the address above.

This book is sold subject to the condition that it shall not,
by way of trade or otherwise, be lent, re-sold, hired out, or otherwise
circulated without the publisher's prior consent in any form of binding
or cover other than that in which it is published and without a similar
condition including this condition being imposed
on the subsequent purchaser.

A catalogue record for this book is available from the British Library

Library of Congress Cataloging in Publication Data
(Available on request)
ISBN 0 19 262303 6 (Hbk)
ISBN 0 19 262302 8 (Pbk)

Typeset by Footnote Graphics, Warminster, Wilts
Printed in Hong Kong

RE
48.2
.C5D48
1994

PREFACE

The aim of this book is to provide the general practitioner and paediatrician with a concise, illustrated clinical guide to eye disorders affecting children. This book provides a broad overview of disorders which may affect the eyes in childhood; further detailed information is available from reference texts already on the market.

Part 1 is an outline of the structure, function, and development of the eye. Part 2 describes salient points in the history and general techniques of examination. Part 3 deals with the detection and causes of poor vision, and Part 4 with the diagnosis and management of squint. Parts 5 and 6 cover the differential diagnosis of common paediatric eye disorders and Part 7 discusses the eye manifestations of systemic disease, the implications of visual handicap for the child and family, and blindness prevention.

It is only for the purposes of convenience and convention that both child and examiner are referred to as 'he' in this book.

Edinburgh   B.D.
January, 1994   G.T.M.

WILLIAM F. MAAG LIBRARY
YOUNGSTOWN STATE UNIVERSITY

ACKNOWLEDGEMENTS

Many of the illustrations in this book are from the teaching collection at the Princess Alexandra Eye Pavilion, and the personal slide collection of Professor A. S. M. Lim. Arthur Lim provided advice and encouragement, and without his generous support this book could not have been produced.

Dr A. Somner kindly allowed us to reproduce illustrations of vitamin A deficiency.

We would like to thank our colleagues in Edinburgh—Dr Hector Chawla, Dr Barry Cullen, and Dr Brian Fleck—they reviewed the manuscript and gave valuable advice.

Finally, special thanks to the staff of the Oxford University Press for their support and encouragement in the production of this book.

CONTENTS

PART ONE

Introduction

Anatomy

Function

Development

Introduction

The general practitioner and paediatrician should be familiar with examining the child's eye, recognizing common eye problems, knowing when to start treatment, and when to refer. Children with eye disorders commonly present to the GP and paediatrician and their skills in ophthalmic diagnosis are the key to successful treatment. The first eye examination should be at birth in order to detect structural abnormalities. Further checks at preschool and school age allow visual assessment, detection of refractive error, amblyopia, squint, and organic eye disease.

The aim of this book is to present a simple approach to the diagnosis of eye disease in childhood. We hope this book will aid all medical and nursing staff in 'the front line' of primary paediatric eye care.

Who is involved?

Parents and grandparents are usually the first to recognize their child's eye problem.

Neonatologists perform the initial postnatal examination.

General practitioners check a child's eye during infancy and again at 3–4 years. They are usually the first port of call for children with an acute eye problem.

Health visitors are involved in vision screening of the preschool child.

School nurses screen vision in school age children.

Hospital paediatricians particularly neurologists may detect eye disease in children with other problems such as cerebral palsy or hydrocephalus.

Community paediatricians assess visual and general development.

Orthoptists work closely with ophthalmologists and are involved in the management of amblyopia and squint.

Opticians or optometrists are skilled in vision assessment and testing for glasses (refraction); dispensing opticians are qualified to provide spectacles.

Ophthalmologists are responsible for the medical and surgical management of all sight-threatening eye diseases but are not usually involved in the primary care of eye disease in children.

Anatomy

The newborn eye closely resembles the adult eye but there are differences. It is smaller in overall dimensions and the outer layers are thinner and more pliable. Growth of the eye continues at a rapid rate in the first year of life and the most rapid period of visual maturation is during the first six months of life.

Eyelids and eyelashes

In their correct positions, the upper lid should just touch the upper aspect of the cornea and the lower lid should lie beneath the lower edge of the cornea. The lashes of the child should be clean, free from crusts, and turn outwards away from the eyeball.

Eyeball and orbit

The conjunctiva is a transparent membrane draping over the exposed surface of the eyeball except the corneal surface. It tucks into the recess behind, and reflects on to the back surfaces of upper and lower eyelids. The lower recess or fornix can be inspected by pulling down the lower lid, and getting the child (by asking or attracting the child's attention) to look up; this exposes the healthy pink, smooth conjunctiva, which readily prolapses forwards. Beneath the conjunctiva is the sclera which forms a tough outer protective coat and shows as the 'white of the eye'. The cornea is the transparent window in front of the coloured iris, and when healthy, reflects light like a bright mirror. The anterior chamber is the space between the iris and cornea, which is filled with watery (aqueous) fluid, and the central aperture of the iris is the pupil. Behind the iris lies the lens of the eye, which is transparent and is suspended by fine ligaments or zonules, which are slung from finger-like projections (ciliary processes). Contraction of the encircling ciliary muscle slackens the tension in the zonule, and the lens assumes a globular shape, while relaxation of the ciliary muscle pulls the zonules taut, stretching the elastic lens into a more discoid shape. The transparent vitreous jelly fills most of the eye behind the lens and the retina covers its inner spherical surface. The lens, vitreous, and retina should transmit a red glow or reflex when reflected light is observed using an ophthalmoscope. The retina consists of neurones and photoreceptors lined externally by a pigmented epithelium and choroid, which in turn is enclosed by a sclera coat. Axons stream across the inner aspect of the retina towards the optic nerve head, and leave the eye through a hiatus in the sclera to form the optic nerve. The nerve is invested by a sheath of dura containing cerebrospinal fluid, which is continuous with the investing coats of the brain. The optic nerves meet at the chiasma where the nasal fibres cross over. Visual information from the temporal field of vision is carried in these fibres. The fibres project to the lateral geniculate ganglion synapse, then radiate to the occipital cortex.

The child's eye: normal anatomy. Reproduced by kind permission of Churchill Livingstone.

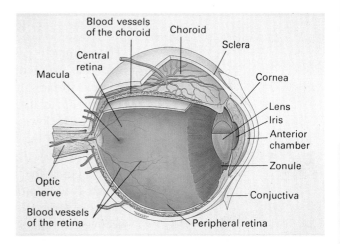

The orbit is the bony cavity which houses and protects the eyeball, connective tissue, and extraocular muscles from the adjacent sinuses and unexpected blows. The lacrimal gland is hidden and protected behind its upper, outer aspect and produces the aqueous component of the tears. Two small holes or puncta, one in each lid drain fluid into the lacrimal sac which is sited deep in a recess next to the nose. The eyeball moves by the action of three pairs of extraocular muscles, each originating from the walls of the orbit and inserted into different sites in the sclera. The horizontal and the vertical recti muscles move the eyes right and left, and up and down respectively and oblique muscles move the eyes along a diagonal path. The muscle pairs act together like reins on a horse, one pulling in, and the other letting out.

WILLIAM F. MAAG LIBRARY
YOUNGSTOWN STATE UNIVERSITY

Function

The integration of tissues with special properties (Table 1.1) allows the eye to fulfil its principal function of vision. Healthy lids and tear flow maintain the anterior corneal surface in a clean and moist state, essential for its optical function.

Table 1.1 Properties and functions of ocular structures

	Special property	Function
Cornea	transparent	optical—fixed focus
Lens	transparent	optical—variable focus
Choroid	vascular	nutrition for retina
Retina	{ light receptors	converts light impulses
	neural elements	to neural message

The optical properties of the eye allow images from variable distances to be focused upon the retina. The images of near objects are focused by a process called accommodation, which is accomplished through the action of the ciliary muscle on the zonule and lens. The neonate has a fixed focus of 20–30 cm, at three months this reaches 75 cm and by six months of age a child can focus from near to infinity. A child unable to focus images from different distances on to the retina has a refractive error. A hypermetropic child sees close objects as a blur, as the image focus lies behind the retina despite maximum accommodative effort. A myopic child sees distant objects as a blur as the image focus lies in front of the retina. Refractive error is discussed in Part 3. The retina converts the image into a neural message through a process called transduction which is mediated by light sensitive pigment in the photoreceptors. Cone photoreceptors serve colour vision under bright illumination, and rod photoreceptors serve achromatic vision in dim illumination. The macula is a small area of the retina, a few millimetres in diameter, sited temporal to the optic nerve head. It contains the highest concentration of photoreceptors, mainly cones, and is responsible for central acuity and colour vision. When the eye fixes on an object straight ahead, it is upon the macula that the image falls. The remaining retina has fewer photoreceptors, mostly rods, and is responsible for the peripheral vision allowing us to perceive objects 'out of the corner' of our eyes.

To ensure synchronized movements of both eyes there is close coordination between corresponding muscle pairs. The midbrain controls eye movements through cranial nerves III (oculomotor), IV (trochlear), and VI (abducens). The eyes are held in parallel alignment in all positions of gaze except during the acts of convergence and divergence, when the eyes see incoming or out-going objects. Rapid visual feedback to the extraocular muscles permits accurate binocular tracking of slowly or rapidly moving targets. Information from the vestibular apparatus and cerebellum is fed to the midbrain, so that fine adjustments can be made to the eye positions to compensate for altered head and body posture.

Development

Prenatal development

The 22-day embryo shows the first signs of eye development and there follows a silent ballet of sliding, folding, and replicating groups of cells. A pair of shallow grooves appear on either side of the invaginating forebrain and form extensions or optic vesicles which lie beneath the surface ectoderm. Invagination of the vesicle produces a central depression and ventral groove along which the hyaloid artery travels to reach the developing lens.

The lips of the choroidal fissure fuse during the seventh week of the embryo's life and the mouth of the optic cup becomes the round aperture of the future pupil. Meanwhile cells of the surface ectoderm elongate to form the lens placode and become pinched off to form a vesicle lying in the mouth of the optic cup. The cells of the posterior wall of the lens vesicle elongate, forming long fibres stretching anteriorly to obliterate the lumen (primary lens fibres) until they reach the anterior wall, to form the nucleus of the lens. Secondary lens fibres from the equator of the lens vesicle are added to the outside of the nucleus in 'onion skin' fashion and this continues throughout life.

A membrane in front of the lens and iris, the iridopupillary membrane, is separated from anterior layers of mesenchyme and surface epithelium by formation of the anterior chamber; it is these layers of mesenchyme that give rise to the cornea. Neural crest cells invade the recess between the iris and cornea and form the trabecular meshwork and drainage apparatus for the aqueous humour.

The anterior segment of the optic cup divides to form the primitive iris and ciliary body. Externally, mesenchyme condenses to form the ciliary muscles which connect to the lens by a circle of elastic fibres, the suspensory ligaments. Contraction of the ciliary muscle

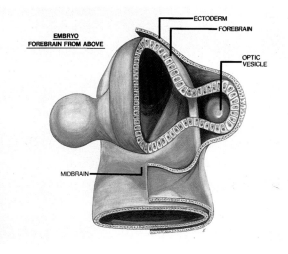

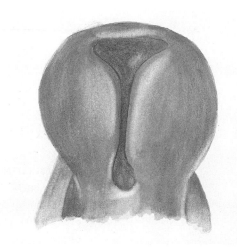

Embryology of the eye. Optic cup forms by invagination. Reproduced by kind permission of Churchill Livingstone.

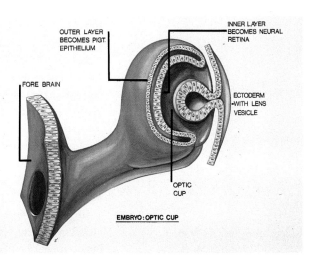

changes the tension in the ligaments and alters the shape and focusing of the lens. The inner layer of the optic cup thickens to form the light receptive elements: the rods and cones, the retinal neurones and supporting cells, and the inner axons of the nerve cells which converge towards the optic stalk, the future optic nerve. The outer layer of the cup becomes pigmented and is the primitive pigment epithelium of the retina.

By the seventh week the choroidal fissure has enclosed the hyaloid artery which is destined to become the central artery of the retina, and nerve fibres from the eye to brain have developed within the optic stalk. The vascularized primary vitreous cavity is replaced by a clear avascular secondary vitreous.

The tissue surrounding the optic cup differentiates into an inner vascularized and pigmented layer (choroid) and an outer layer (sclera) which is continuous anteriorly with the cornea and posteriorly with the dura mater surrounding the optic nerve. Axons grow as the optic nerve from the retina towards the chiasm and myelination continues postnatally.

Visual maturation

Maturation of the eye and visual pathway continues during early childhood. The photoreceptors assume a longer and thinner shape and their function progressively improves. Complex neurophysiological modelling occurring in the higher visual pathways allows the construction of a single three dimensional image from the visual input of two eyes. When looking at an object, each retina is presented with a similar, though slightly different image because of the separation between the eyes. The subtly disparate images stimulate corresponding points in the retinas of the two eyes, which are fused to a single stereoscopic image in the brain. The correct alignment of the eyes is critical, otherwise confusing information is fed to the visual pathway. The binocular vision reflex maintains the correct alignment of the eyes, and is normally present by six months of age.

In the presence of a structurally normal eye and visual pathway, certain prerequisites must be met in order to achieve optimal visual function in each eye.

For both eyes to work binocularly a sharp, formed image must fall on corresponding points on each retina. If this does not occur, optimal central visual acuity does not develop; the binocular reflex should maintain the parallel alignment of the eyes otherwise the visual signal to the deviating eye is 'switched off'. These changes are reversible within certain time limits, after which the visual system has matured and is inflexible and amblyopia or a 'lazy' eye is the result (Part 3). The critical period in visual development during which re-modelling is possible is not clearly defined but is thought to be during the first years of life, though amblyopia may be at least partly reversible until eight or nine years of age.

Abnormal development

Abnormal development leads to a spectrum of structural defects. *Coloboma* is a failure of fusion of the choroidal fissure during the seventh week of development. Usually the iris is involved but the defect may extend into the ciliary body, retina, choroid, and optic nerve. *Microphthalmos* is a small eye associated with other ocular abnormalities.

Persistent pupillary membrane is an innocuous remnant of the iridopupillary membrane. *Persistent hyperplastic primary vitreous* leads to an opaque mass behind the lens and poor vision (Part 3). *Cataract* is a lens which becomes opaque during intrauterine life. The lens is most actively differentiating during the sixth week of life when the primary lens fibres are elongating and it is at this stage that it is most vulnerable to interference. Maternal rubella and other viruses, vitamin deficiency, hypothyroidism, and irradiation are cataractogenic factors (Part 3). *Glaucoma* results from insufficient drainage of aqueous humour and is caused by malformation of the drainage angle. This condition may be acquired genetically and can be associated with other iris and corneal malformations. Absence of the iris apart from a peripheral frill is called *aniridia* and this condition is often associated with glaucoma (Part 5). *Optic nerve hypoplasia* is seen in association with midline brain defects, for example septo-optic dysplasia in association with endocrine abnormalities. The optic nerve

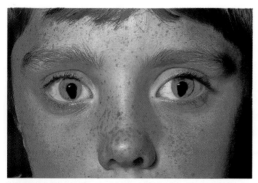

Iris coloboma indicates incomplete closure of the
fetal cleft.

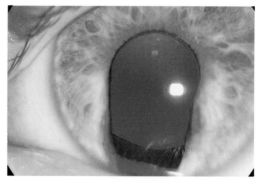

Iris coloboma showing a sector defect in the iris.

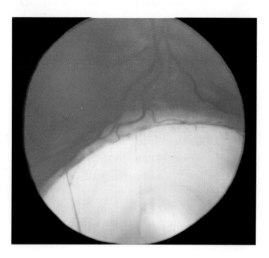

Choroidal coloboma. Crescentic absence of choroid
causes a corresponding field defect.

looks one-third to one-half its normal size and can lead
to a wide range of visual dysfunction.

Craniofacial dysostosis is failure in the development of
the primitive mesoderm in formation of the skull
bones. If premature fusion of the skull sutures occurs
whilst the brain is still expanding, eye and neurological
problems may occur during childhood (Parts 3 and 6).

The developing eye is susceptible to infection by
rubella, toxoplasmosis, cytomegalovirus and syphilis
during the first trimester. Drugs such as anticonvulsants
and alcohol also impair ocular development. Infection
acquired maternally causes inflammation, opacifica-
tion, and scarring of the cornea, lens, or retina; microphthalmos may also be present. Toxic agents may cause
global ocular malformations for example microphthalmos, coloboma, and optic nerve hypoplasia.

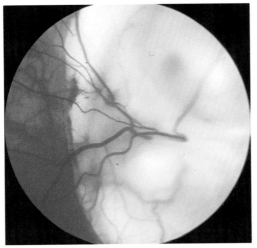

Choroidal coloboma involving optic nerve causing profound visual loss.

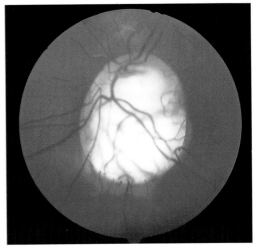

Coloboma affecting the optic nerve.

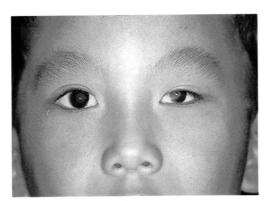

Microphthalmos. A small left eye and corneal scar reflects developmental failure of the whole eye.

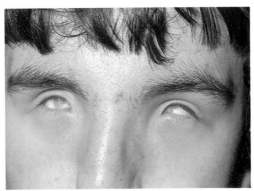

Bilateral microphthalmos.

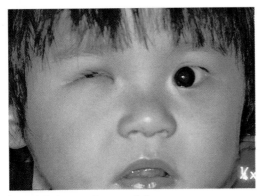

Anophthalmos – absence of the eye.

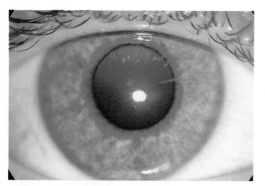

(a) Persistent pupillary membrane. Fine strand bridges the pupil but causes no visual impairment.

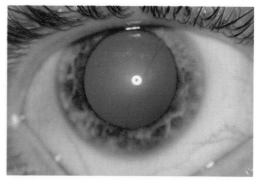

(b) A fine strand is attached to the iris.

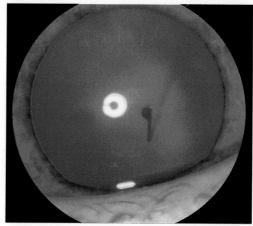

(c) Persistent hyaloid artery stretches from the posterior lens to the optic nerve head, and causes no visual impairement.

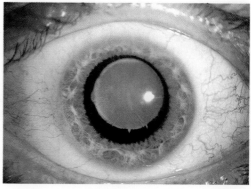

Cataract.

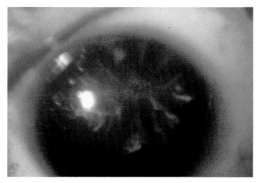

Aniridia. The iris is absent exposing the white star-shaped cataract.

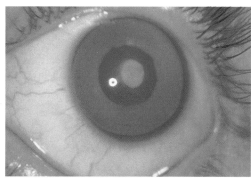

Aniridia with central circular cataract.

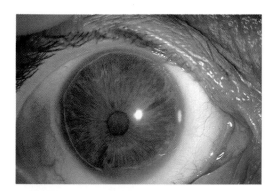

Axenfeld's anomaly. Peripheral iris is adherent to the cornea appearing as a white ring. Glaucoma is associated.

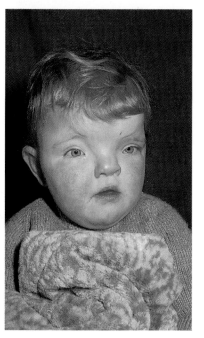

Craniofacial dysostosis with hypertelorism.

(a) Toxoplasmosis has destroyed an area of retina
and choroid exposing the underlying white sclera.
(b) Blood vessels within the scar are choroidal and
are not continuous with the retinal circulation.

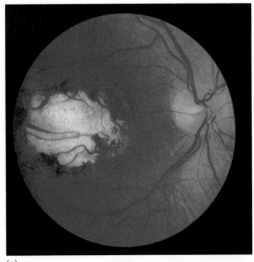

(a)

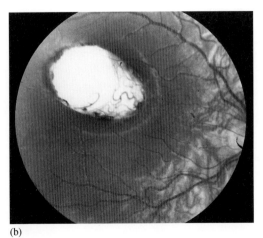

(b)

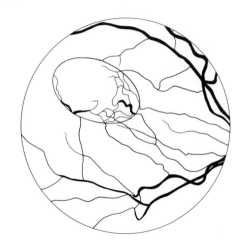

PART TWO

History

Examination

History

The value of the history, usually taken from the mother or grandmother, should never be underestimated. It is an obvious fact that young children are unable to articulate their problem, and will neglect unilateral painless visual deterioration. It is the behaviour of the child which raises suspicion of eye disease. Disinterest in near work or watching television with 'the nose up against the screen' are suggestive of a need for glasses. Persistent eye rubbing may be a sign of ocular allergy and reluctance to open the eyes in daylight suggests photophobia. These clues are useful and should be sought from the history. The child should be observed during the history taking and any signs documented. The examination begins as soon as the child enters the room and each piece of information should be recognized and noted. A child usually refuses to submit to a stepwise examination and will often reveal his symptoms and signs in a disorderly sequence which are later fitted together like a jig-saw puzzle into a final diagnostic picture.

In order to gather information about the child's eye problem, it is valuable to ask who first noticed the symptom, what it was and when it became apparent. Other questions which should be asked are: What is the effect on the child's behaviour? Is it unilateral or bilateral? Is it progressive? Further enquiry should cover the child's general health and current medications. Information about the family and the child's birth is also valuable:

● Family history and consanguinity
Although refractive error and squint often run in families they do not follow strict Mendelian principles. Other diseases affecting the eye such as cataract, glaucoma, retinal dystrophies, and optic atrophy may be inherited.

• Perinatal infection

Congenitally acquired rubella, cytomegalovirus, and toxoplasmosis could now be joined by human immunodeficiency virus (HIV) in causing sight-threatening eye disease.

• Postnatal history

Low birth weight and prematurity are associated with a wide spectrum of eye disorders such as retinopathy of prematurity, refractive error, and squint.

Asking general questions allows understanding of the eye complaint in the context of the child's overall development and background. Relevant areas to be covered are the mental and physical developmental milestones—delay in development or associated disability should be noted—and social conditions—social and emotional deprivation with unexplained eye injuries should raise the possibility of child abuse.

Information concerning the visual behaviour of a child may be gleaned by enquiring about the child's response to his surroundings. Normal milestones are shown in Table 2.1. Other features concerning visual behaviour should be noted, particularly school activities as detailed in Table 2.2. A searching enquiry may unearth more subtle visual problems, for instance a

Table 2.1 The development of normal visual behaviour

Responsive smiling	first weeks
Fixes upon bright light	3 weeks
Follows objects	3 months
Looks for toys	1 year
Looks at pictures	18 months
Recognizes adults	2 years

Table 2.2 Symptoms of refractive error

Myopia
Books held close
Unable to see the board in class
Poor performance in outdoor games
Eyelids squeezed when looking into the distance
Associated divergent squint (Part 4)

Hypermetropia
Difficulty reading
Associated convergent squint (Part 4)

child who confuses coloured pens, foods, or street and car lights may have colour vision deficiency. The child who becomes distressed or clumsy in dim light may have retinitis pigmentosa (Part 3).

Further enquiry during the history-taking may now be directed to specific details concerning the presenting complaint. For example, if the eye is red, ask if there has been discharge, which suggests infection. If the child has periorbital bruising, ask about recent trauma. Altered behaviour may have an ocular cause, for example persistent eye-rubbing, habitual eye squeezing, and rapid eye blinking in a child with lid infection or allergy. Although one symptom is likely to be most prominent, usually there are a combination of symptoms and signs, for example redness and discharge in a child with bacterial conjunctivitis (Part 5), or the sinister combination of **white pupil** and squint in a child with retinoblastoma (Part 3). The significance of common eye complaints in children are described below, and are adddressed in more detail later in the book.

The conjunctiva becomes **red** either because inflammation leads to dilation of the blood vessels, or because of underlying haemorrhage. Most infective and allergic external eye diseases inflame the conjunctiva, and the tortuous angry vessels confer a diffuse bright redness to this normally opalescent tissue. Even minor trauma can rupture the delicate conjunctival vessels, allowing a well circumscribed collection of blood. Possible causes of a mucopurulent **discharge** include bacterial conjunctivitis, keratitis, and ophthalmia neonatorum. The sticky quality of the discharge can make lid opening difficult. (Bathing the lids permits the lids to be opened). Excessive watering or tearing accompanies allergic and viral conditions of the external eye. Chronic **watering** indicates a blocked tear duct. A subtarsal foreign body produces intense local irritation with watering. Acute bilateral **irritation** of the eyelids is usually due to allergy; chronic infection of the eyelids induces persistent itching and eye-rubbing (Part 6). The **photophobic** child shies away from bright lights, squeezes both eyes tightly and shields or hides his face away from the light. When exposed to light, if there is accompanying watering and distress, glaucoma should be suspected (Part 5). Corneal disease, albinism, migraine, and meningitis are other causes of photo-phobia. Light-sensitivity is also present in children with divergent squint and they tend to close the squinting eye in bright sunlight (Part 4). The ocular causes of **headache** and eye fatigue include uncorrected refractive error and latent squint. It should be remembered that headache is also a symptom of migraine, meningitis, and raised intracranial pressure.

Unusual appearances in the position and movement of a child's eyes or head may prompt the parents to seek attention; it is the doctor's responsibility to decide if the 'odd' appearance is clinically significant. A mother may describe a variety of eye symptoms such as squeezing or screwing the eyelids as a 'squint'. A true **squint** is an in-turning or out-turning eye, which can be associated with poor vision or lack of the binocular reflex; the angle of eye non-alignment is constant in all directions of gaze (Part 4). If the angle of the squint is not constant in all positions of gaze and is only apparent when the child looks in a particular direction, this may be due to an ocular muscle palsy (Part 4). A child with this may adopt a **compensatory head posture** viewing the world with head turned and chin elevated or de-pressed. The adopted posture is a tactic to avoid double vision as the eyes are turned in the direction which holds the visual axes straight. Children labelled as suf-fering with 'primary torticollis' with occult eye motility disorders have erroneously undergone surgery to a neck rather than an eye muscle! A drooping upper eyelid or **ptosis** means that either the innervation, or the muscle which elevates the lid is at fault (Parts 4 and 6). If the lid covers the pupillary area, the vision is in jeopardy and this requires swift treatment to prevent permanent visual impairment. A chin up head posture is adopted by children with bilateral ptosis in order to peer through their narrowed palpebral apertures. A tumour seated deep in the orbit can push the eyeball out of position, and this is called **proptosis** (Part 6). The eye may also be displaced in a lateral, superior, or inferior position, and this may shed light upon the site and nature of the space occupying mass. Craniofacial anomalies may be associated with shallow orbits and proptosis. A larger than normal eye may appear promi-nent, caused by glaucoma, progressive myopia, or congenitally enlarged cornea. Parents may notice **roving eye movements** in their child during the early weeks of life which can be normal. If this persists poor vision should be suspected (Part 3). Oscillatory movements of the eyes or **nystagmus** may be a sign of neurological disease (Part 3).

Examination

An overall impression of a child's visual behaviour may be gleaned by noting their reaction to the surroundings and their steadiness of gaze as they enter the room for examination. Abnormal appearances of the head, bruising of the lids, ocular malpositions, or red and watering eyes may be striking features as soon as the child and parent enter the room. It is helpful to compare one side with the other to detect signs of eye disease. Some signs such as a compensatory head posture, facial asymmetry, lid malposition, and pupil size inequalities may be subtle but significant and therefore should never be ignored. The examiner should start with the tests which cause least disturbance to the child, and once the confidence of the child has been won, success in the more difficult aspects of examination is likely.

Visual acuity

After gaining an initial impression of the child during the history taking, an attempt should always be made to perform a test of the essential function of the eye-vision. Visual acuity testing is a measure of macula function and therefore central vision. Quantification of visual acuity can be achieved by using letter or picture charts in children aged 3 years and upwards. Testing visual acuity should be the first step of any eye examination, but can easily be forgotten in the rush to attend to the eye problem. Each eye should be tested in turn, by covering the other. The tests of visual acuity are discussed in Part 3.

Visual field testing

Visual field abnormalities may be due to disease of the retina, optic nerve, or further along the visual pathway (Part 3).

Colour vision

Children with colour vision abnormalities are usually detected by screening. This may be assessed in the older child using colour designs arranged such that a child with colour vision abnormality will fail to recognize specific patterns (Part 3).

Symmetry and structure

The maximum amount of information concerning eye structure and symmetry can be gathered by performing the tests which are least disturbing to the child first. The child's attention span and state of well-being dictate the length of examination. Practice and gentle handling allow a swift and successful eye examination in a well-rested and well-fed child. The position of the lids relative to the eyeball provides information concerning lid function, eye size, and eye position. If the disorder affects one side more than the other comparison between the eyes permits swift detection. The upper lid of one eye may cover more cornea and iris detail than the other in a child with ptosis. An eye which protrudes forwards and exposes more sclera than the other eye is proptosed, although this may give the false impression of an enlarged eye. Abnormal enlargement of the eye, which occurs in childhood glaucoma, will have increased corneal and iris diameter, whereas a microphthalmic eye will have a reduced corneal and iris

Table 2.3 Abnormalities of eye symmetry and structure

Symmetry	Abnormality
Eyelids	Ptosis
Eyeball position	Proptosis
Eye alignment	Squint
Pupil shape	Uveitis
Pupil size	III nerve palsy
	Horner's syndrome
Pupil reactions	Optic nerve disease
Structure	
Eyeball size	Microphthalmos
Corneal diameter	Buphthalmos
Corneal clarity	Ulcer
	Hurler's syndrome
Iris	Coloboma
Fundus reflex	Tumour, cataract

diameter. Closer attention to the pupil may reveal subtle signs, such as a white pupil in an eye with retinoblastoma, an irregular pupil in an eye with uveitis, or a sluggishly reacting pupil to light in an eye with disease of the retina or optic nerve. Table 2.3 is a checklist for examination of the eye and surrounding structures. (The signs referred to in the table are discussed elsewhere in the book.)

Squint

The visual axis is a theoretical line connecting the fixation object with the macula, and a squint exists when the visual axes do not intersect at the point of fixation. A convergent squint exists when one visual axis is turned in, and a divergent squint when one visual axis turns outwards. The angle between the visual axes gives a measure of the size of the squint. The presence of a squint (strabismus) is assessed by examining the corneal light reflexes, testing eye movements, and performing the cover test (Part 4). A concomitant or nonparalytic squint is present in all directions of gaze and is by far the most common type of squint encountered in general practice (Part 4). A noncomitant or paralytic squint is present only when the child looks in the direction of the paretic muscle (Part 4).

Pupils

During the first two months of life, especially if born prematurely, the pupils are often small and react poorly to light. The pupils of a full term infant, however, should react to a direct light stimulus. It is important to use a bright torch light with dim room illumination, and to repeat the test several times to obtain accurate and reliable information. The technique of testing pupil reactions is discussed in Part 3.

Corneal clarity

The healthy cornea reflects the pentorch light like a mirror; however, with disease this normally bright reflective quality of the cornea is lost. Corneal enlargement occurs in childhood glaucoma and corneal clouding is

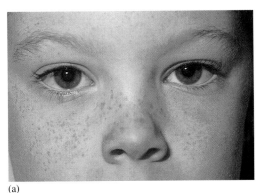 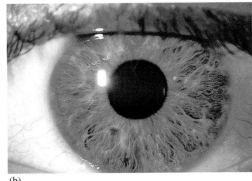

(a)   (b)

Corneal light reflex. The healthy cornea reflects light like a mirror (b) and if the visual axes are parallel the light reflexes fall close to the centre of the pupils (a).

observed in children with certain types of mucopolysaccharidosis. Corneal trauma or ulcer is caused by damage to the superficial epithelial cell layer resulting in a low denuded crater, bare of its protective cover. Despite this breach the cornea still looks quite transparent but the defect is easily seen when orange fluorescein dye is instilled, which is taken up by the abraded area and stains green. Infection of the deeper corneal layers appear as white, ragged opacities, with strands of adherent mucopus and a very red eye (Part 5). Corneal scarring is the long term result, and if the pupillary area is involved sight is seriously affected.

Intraocular pressure

Fluid in the eye is constantly produced and drained. If there is a blockage in the egress of fluid from the eye, the build up of pressure forces fluid into the cornea, which becomes stretched, waterlogged, and cloudy. The corneal diameter, and indeed the whole eye expands, and this sign is called buphthalmos (ox eye). This is discussed further in Part 5.

Anterior chamber

Blood (following trauma) or pus (with severe infection) gravitates to the bottom of the anterior chamber, forming a fluid layer between the iris and cornea (Part 5). Blood in the anterior chamber is called a hyphaema, whereas pus is white and is called a hypopyon. Movement of the eye and head stirs up these collections, and the swirling turbid fluids can produce a diffuse haze which obscures the iris and pupil detail.

A cooperative child may allow the examiner close enough to use a low power magnifying lens for a more detailed examination of the cornea, anterior chamber, iris, and pupil. The lens is held between the thumb and forefinger of one hand and the pentorch in the other hand, to provide oblique illumination. The parent or assistant gently part the lids, though if dextrous, the examiner may be able to do this using both ring fingers.

Ophthalmoscopy

This is the difficult part of the examination; the usual reward for a great deal of effort is a glimpse of a few retinal vessels whilst the elusive optic nerve head remains hidden from view! Using very simple means useful information concerning clarity of the cornea, lens, and vitreous can be gleaned. Babies permit ophthalmoscopy provided the examiner is gentle and patient. The child should be comfortable, for example on the mother's lap or in her arms and infants may find it comforting to suck on a dummy or bottle. The examiner should first ensure that the ophthalmoscope produces a bright and circular beam. The room lights should be dimmed but not switched off completely as the child may panic in the dark. The examiner should then attempt to elicit a retinal reflex by viewing the fundus from a distance of 25–40 cm with no magnification, or, the examiner's refractive error in the aperture of the ophthalmoscope (by rotating the lens rack). The unique transparent quality of the cornea, lens, and vitreous permit the red reflex from the retina to be seen. If dense opacities are present in the cornea, lens, vitreous, and retina, they are seen as silhouettes against a red background. A grey/yellow or white reflex suggests disease in the lens, vitreous, or retina (Part 3). This sign should *never* be missed as the eye may harbour a life-threatening tumour, and a child displaying this sign needs urgent referral to an ophthalmologist. In order to view the disc and central retina the examiner must be especially calm and patient. If the child is afraid of the examination, it may help to demonstrate the procedure on the parent or assistant. An older child may be en-

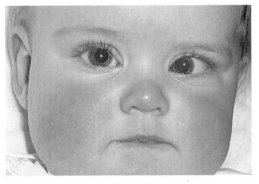

Red reflex in a child with a left convergent squint.

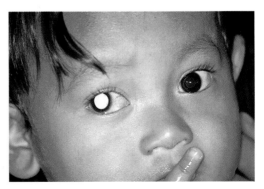

White fundus reflex. The child has a retinoblastoma.

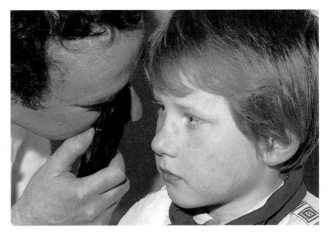

Direct ophthalmoscopy: a skill requiring practice, in order to examine the child's disc and retina

couraged to cooperate by suggesting that they might see a favourite cartoon character through their end of the ophthalmoscope! If the examiner has no refractive error, or if he chooses to wear spectacles, the 0 lens in the ophthalmoscope is chosen, otherwise the appropriate lens is selected. The examiner's right eye should be used for observing the child's right eye, and the left eye for the child's left eye. If necessary, the lids may be gently prised apart using the thumb and forefinger which frees the other hand to hold an ophthalmoscope. Direct ophthalmoscopy confirms the presence of a red reflex though it is of limited value in discerning retinal detail especially in the restless child with undilated pupils. In this situation it is helpful to dilate the pupils; this also permits examination of the peripheral retina.

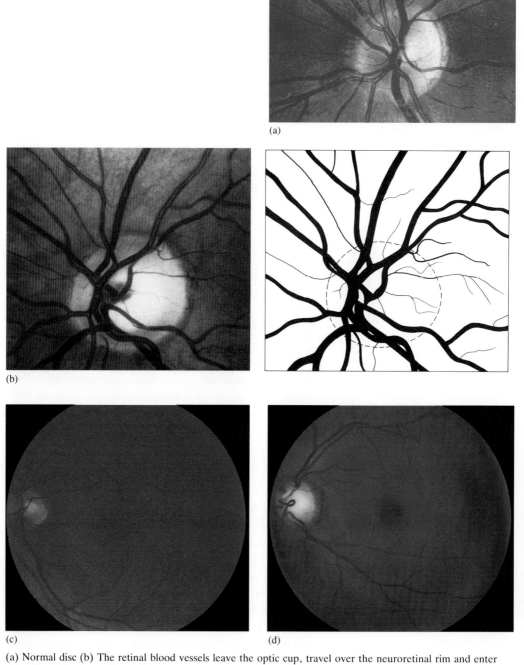

(a)

(b)

(c)   (d)

(a) Normal disc (b) The retinal blood vessels leave the optic cup, travel over the neuroretinal rim and enter the retina. The dotted line indicates the edge of the optic nerve head.
Normal fundus (c). A lightly pigmented fundus of a Caucasian child compared to the more heavily pigmented fundus of an Indian child (d).

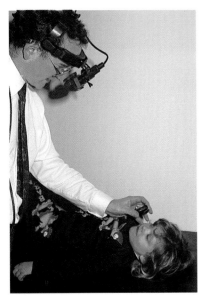

Indirect ophthalmoscopy: this instrument provides a wider view of the retina and is used by eye specialists.

Short acting mydriatics such as tropicamide 0.5% are safe and effective. Precipitating an attack of angle closure glaucoma by dilating the pupils does not occur in children and should not deter the examiner.

Examining a distressed child with an eye problem can be a daunting prospect, though with gentle handling most children allow eye examination. Constant encouragement, coaxing, and even bribery, facilitate cooperation. The examiner may decide to defer eye examination till another day; if the child has an urgent eye problem immediate referral to an eye specialist is the only option.

PART THREE

Poor vision

Poor vision

Visual loss results from occlusion of the pupil, for example by ptosis, or occurs from disease of the cornea, lens, or retina. Associated features such as a red eye, lid bruising, squint, or altered visual behaviour may bring the child to medical attention. However, poor vision may remain undetected, particularly if only one eye is affected, or if the eyes are white and without other ocular signs.

Detecting poor vision

Observation of the normal child will establish a record of the expected actions and responses to visual stimuli and surroundings. Success in examination depends on some cooperation from the child. To achieve this the examiner must attract and hold the interest of the child and gain his confidence from the outset. The visual system of a child must be examined in accordance with his age and ability; the examination can only be as complete as the age and stage allows. In order to test the vision in each eye, an effective cover is required. If the vision in one eye is thought to be poor, testing their better eye first will allow the child to become familiar and confident with the procedure. An infant with poor eyesight in one eye will tearfully resent occlusion of the better eye. Quantifying the level of vision is difficult in young children and more reliable information can be obtained as the baby grows as described below. Simple and inexpensive tests of vision are described below.

Visual assessment in infants

Evidence that a child can see is reassuring to parents. The newborn infant is able to close his eyes when bright light falls on them, and mimics facial expression from the first day of life. Eye to eye contact, responsive smiling in early life, watching light through a window or from an electric bulb are valuable clues that the infant can see.

Fixing and following

In early life, a mother's face is a potent stimulus for this response, and later a pentorch or small brightly coloured toys can be used.

Pupillary responses

Direct and consensual light reactions provide some indirect clues regarding neonatal vision. Although the pupils may be small in the first few months of life, a response to a bright light stimulus in the older child suggests intact optic nerve pathways and this is discussed below 'page 52'.

Suppression of nystagmus

Nystagmus may be physiologically induced and observed in a fellow passenger looking out of a window in a train or bus. This form of rhythmic eye oscillation, called nystagmus, can also be induced by bodily rotation, and this is the basis of the test. The infant is held firmly in the observer's arms so that each faces the other and good eye contact is established. The observer explains to the parents that he is going to spin round suddenly while watching the baby's eye movements, and then performs this rotation, stopping abruptly after one revolution. The normal baby will show two or three beats of nystagmus and then gaze steadily at the observer; however, the baby with bilaterally impaired vision will continue to show nystagmus for several seconds.

Visual assessment in older children

In order to quantify visual acuity, standard test charts are used to test both distance and near vision. Children over the age of 3 years generally cooperate with these tests providing the child does not become bored or distracted. Therefore, constant encouragement should be given. If an uncooperative child is wary of the examiner, a parent can be encouraged to participate though should not give the child inadvertent clues. Variations of the Snellen chart using symbols, pictures,

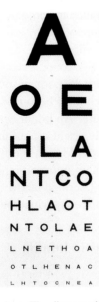

Snellen chart. The distance visual acuity is an expression of the lowest line of letters recognized at a certain distance from the eye.

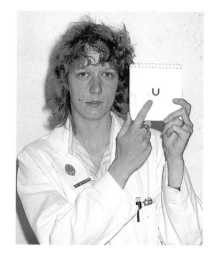

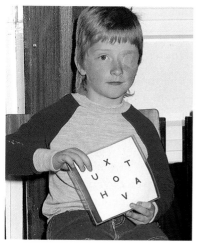

Sheridan Gardiner cards. Pictures or letters may be used to test visual acuity. Each eye is tested in turn, and the child correctly identifies the letter presented to him.

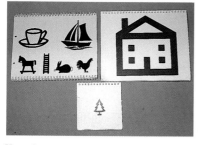

Kay pictures.

or letters of distinctive shape make the same principle available to younger children, and an accurate test can be made from about thirty months of age. The visual acuity should be tested in each eye separately, by always covering the other with a piece of card— covering an eye with a hand invites the possibility of peeking through gaps between the fingers! The distance between the test card and child should be 6 metres (or through a mirror at 3 metres), and there are a range of sizes of the test stimulus. The largest figure is so large that it is seen by a normal eye at 60 m and if this is the only figure seen the visual acuity is recorded as 6/60. The next largest test stimulus presented is seen by the normal eye at 36 metres—if this is the smallest figure seen the acuity is recorded as 6/36. The child with normal vision can see the 6 metre test card and some-times even smaller stimuli recorded as 6/5 or 6/4.

The E test may be used to test the visual acuity of preschool age children (under five years old). The child is placed before a chart bearing numerous figures of the letter E in different sizes and orientation. The examiner points to each figure on the chart, and the child, hold-ing a reference card cut in the shape of an E, orientates this to match the figure. The child who does not see the figure may try and guess at the orientation, though this is usually obvious by the child's behaviour during the examination. Other tests which employ a reference chart are Kay pictures and the Sheridan Gardiner test. The standard Snellen chart may be used to test the vision of school age children if they are familiar with letters of the alphabet. A child with poor vision due to refractive error will be able to see more clearly through a pinhole, which may be easily fashioned using a piece of card. Reading tests are also available for use with older children. If long distance vision is good and near vision poor, the child is likely to be long-sighted or hypermetropic, but if long distance vision is poor and near vision good, he is short-sighted or myopic.

Causes of poor visual acuity

Common and preventable causes of poor vision in childhood include refractive error and the so-called 'lazy' eye or amblyopia.

Refractive error

Refractive error means that the eye cannot produce a sharply focused image of an object on the retina, resulting in a blurred view. This is an optical problem and in most instances is correctable with spectacle lenses. Older children with uncorrected refractive errors may be found to squeeze their eyelids when looking at a distant object, peer at them sideways, hold their books too close, or be disinterested in near work altogether! A young child is unable to provide a verbal response to a letter chart, and therefore requires an objective refraction test. The optical error may be determined by first neutralizing the accommodative power of the eye by using topical atropine 1%, and then observing reflections from a streak of light shone into the eye.

Hypermetropia

A long-sighted or hypermetropic eye cannot focus on near objects accurately without the help of an additional converging or convex lens. Low degrees of hypermetropia can be overcome through accommodative effort. Accommodation and convergence are closely linked reflexes, which may become disrupted in the hypermetropic child, who overconverges in a vain attempt to overcome inadequate accommodation. Consequently, a common presentation of hypermetropia in a young child is an associated convergent squint (see Part 4).

Myopia

A short-sighted or myopic eye cannot focus on distant objects without the use of a diverging or concave lens. A common presentation of myopia is an adolescent who has difficulty seeing the board in class. The onset and progression of myopia usually occurs during adolescence.

Astigmatism

An astigmatic eye sees far and near objects as a blur because the focusing power of the cornea varies according to the meridian in which the light rays pass into the

Hypermetropia
The rays of light converge behind the retina

Hypermetropia with convex lens
The rays of light are now focused on the retina

Hypermetropes without convex glasses see objects near to the eye out of focus and may overconverge to compensate—this exacerbates a convergent squint

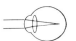

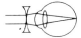

Myopia
The rays of light converge in front of the retina

Myopia with concave lens
The rays of light are focused on the retina

Myopes without concave glasses see distant objects out of focus and may overdiverge to compensate— this exacerbates a divergent squint.

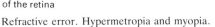

Refractive error. Hypermetropia and myopia.

Association between refractive error and squint.

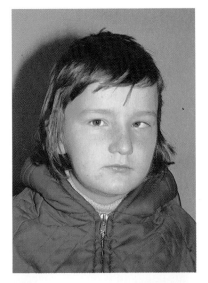

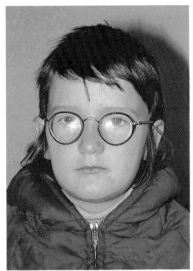

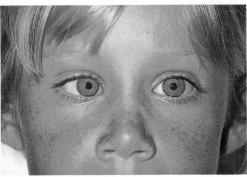

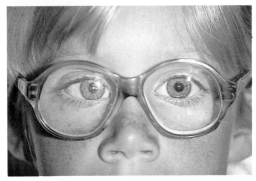

Convergent squint. Correction of the refractive error with glasses improves both the vision and cosmetic appearance in these 2 boys.

eye. A lens which has power in only one plane is required to rectify the problem.

If the two eyes have a very different refractive error (anisometropia) problems can arise with simultaneous perception of the two images, as one is inevitably blurred. This can be difficult to treat as a child may not be able to tolerate large differences in lens powers because of the disparity in magnification (and therefore image sizes) between the two eyes. Contact lenses produce an almost normal sized image and may be the solution for some children.

Young children with suspected refractive error should always be referred to an ophthalmologist who can check for amblyopia, squint, and other eye disease in addition to performing a refraction test. In the absence of other eye disease, ophthalmic opticians or optometrists are best placed to carry out vision checks, refract, and prescribe glasses for the older child. Optometrists are highly skilled in vision testing, refraction, and basic eye examination.

Amblyopia

Amblyopia is a term used for a poorly seeing eye in which no organic lesion is detected and implies a deprivation of formed visual stimulus, an abnormality of binocular interaction or both. Up to 5 per cent of the general population are affected. Refractive error and amblyopia are common, easily identified, and can be treated cheaply and effectively. It is a painless sight-threatening condition, which often occurs unilaterally, usually presents late, and is only discovered on routine testing or when a coexisting strabismus (squint) draws attention to the problem. Amblyopia is associated with squint (commonly convergent), visual deprivation, for example delayed treatment of ptosis or cataract, or excessive hypermetropia and unequal refractive errors. The earlier amblyopia is detected the more successful the treatment will be. Children with amblyopia should be referred to an ophthalmologist, who can confirm the diagnosis, exclude other eye disease, and initiate therapy.

Treatment of amblyopia by occlusion therapy is supervised by both ophthalmologist and orthoptist.

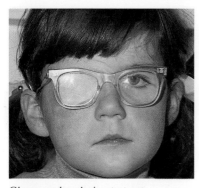

Occlusion therapy to treat an amblyopic right eye, therefore the left eye is occluded.

Glasses and occlusion to treat amblyopia in a hypermetropic child.

Any refractive error is eliminated with glasses, and causes of visual deprivation treated prior to occlusion. Placing a patch over the normal fixing eye for several hours each day whilst vision is stimulated will force the amblyopic eye to work, though close supervision is vital lest the normal eye become amblyopic through stimulus deprivation.

Poor colour vision

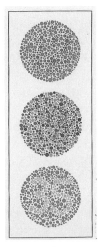

Colour vision test.

An older child may show colour confusion when looking at colour television, foods, or car lights, though colour vision abnormality is often first detected at routine screening. Hereditary colour vision anomalies are common and acquired causes are rare. The former is an X-linked disorder, affecting 6 per cent of males in the West and is usually colour confusion between red and green. Career choices are influenced by such defects, for example normal colour vision is a requirement for some occupations in the UK Armed Forces. Acquired colour vision abnormality may be a sign of retina or optic nerve disorder—colours appear 'washed out', and there is loss of colour intensity.

Bilateral poor vision from birth

Parents will usually show concern if their child fails to show signs of visual attention by looking and following objects by four months of age, though he may be responsive to sounds. Although the visual system is relatively mature at birth, myelination of the optic nerves is a postnatal process, and if prolonged may lead to delayed visual maturation. The diagnosis is made after excluding other causes of blindness in infancy and spontaneous visual improvement occurs. The mother is usually the first person to suspect that her child cannot see and she may have noticed altered visual behaviour, abnormal eye movements, or photophobia. Relevant questions in the history taking should be, is there a family history of eye disease and are the parents related to each other? Recessive genes are responsible for a host of eye disorders. Was the child born prematurely and with low birth weight? Prematurity and anoxia or hyperoxia cause retinal and neuroophthalmic disorders. Examination should begin with an assessment of general physical and mental development. Structural eye defects may be obvious, for example coloboma or microphthalmia. Are there neuroophthalmic signs? If nystagmus is present is it symmetrical, jerky, pendular, vertical, horizontal, or a combination? Does the child fix and follow and are the pupil reactions abnormal? Does the fundus examination show a white reflex? The differential diagnosis of an apparently blind infant would include cataract, glaucoma, aniridia, albinism, high refractive error, retinopathy of prematurity, optic nerve abnormality, or cerebral damage. The child should be referred promptly to an eye specialist where further investigations can be performed. This would include tests of visual function.

Optokinetic nystagmus is a vision-mediated, physiological reflex which can be induced by rotating a black and white striped drum (Catford drum) before the infant. This reflex is normally present from six weeks of age and gives a crude estimate of vision. The standard drum with spots or stripes parallel to the axis of rotation is used to elicit nystagmus in the child. A variation made from a series of squares on a broad tape is more convenient to use and carry about. Preferential looking is a behavioural assessment of visual acuity and relies on the child's preference for looking at a striped pattern rather than a grey background. This test is available in eye units, but in the future it may have a place in the general practitioner's surgery. Electrodiagnostic tests are necessarily more elaborate and require complex electronic recording, stimulating equipment, and technical staff. The visually evoked potential (VEP) tests the integrity of the cerebrum as well as the anterior visual pathway. The computer generated pattern evokes a cortical potential which may be measured using scalp electrodes. The absence of a response in the early months of life does not necessarily indicate visual handicap. Visual maturation may be delayed without any residual deficit. A positive response is an optimistic sign.

A more detailed examination of the child can be carried out under general anaesthesia in order to evaluate both eyes fully. This permits measurement of the corneal diameter and intraocular pressure, examination of the filtration angle and retina, and if the retina can-

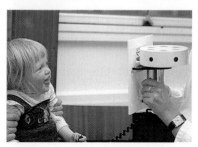

Catford drum. An electronically driven oscillating spot can test vision. If the spot is seen, the child's eye follows. After introducing the instrument to the child, each eye is tested separately.

not be seen, an ultrasound scan of the eye may be performed.

Leukocoria

Usually, a 'white pupil' is first noticed by the child's parents, and a constant convergent or divergent squint may also be present. The diagnosis of a child with leukocoria is retinoblastoma until proven otherwise, and urgent ophthalmic referral is mandatory.

Retinoblastoma

Retinoblastoma, a malignant tumour of the retina, occurs spontaneously as a somatic mutation or by dominant inheritance. It usually arises in the first three years of life, and is fairly advanced when either leukocoria or squint is first detected. Other late presenting features may be hyphaema, the red and painful eye of glaucoma, or orbital inflammation. Although irradiation can be used to treat small tumours, removal (enucleation) of the eye is often necessary. The ophthalmologist must exclude other diseases affecting the vitreous and retina which may present as leukocoria and simulate retinoblastoma, for example intraocular infection, cataract, and retinopathy of prematurity.

Toxocara

Toxocara infestation tends to present as leukocoria in the older child who has close contact with puppies or other animals. Toxocara is a parasitic nematode found in cat and dog faeces which can infest the eye causing intense intraocular inflammation, which may respond to systemic steroids, though the visual outlook is poor. A detailed history, family history, and examination under anaesthesia usually allows the ophthalmologist to distinguish between retinoblastoma and the other causes of leukocoria.

Congenital cataract

Congenital cataract is occasionally caused by rubella, or it may be the first sign of a metabolic disorder,

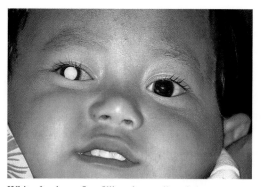

White fundus reflex filling the pupil and the eye.

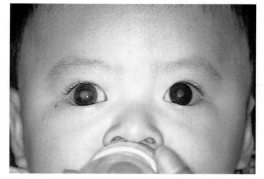

Grey fundus reflex in both eyes in a child with bilateral retinoblastoma.

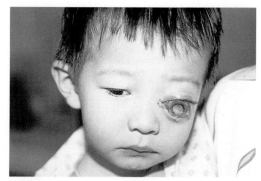

White fundus reflex and proptosis in late presenting retinoblastoma.

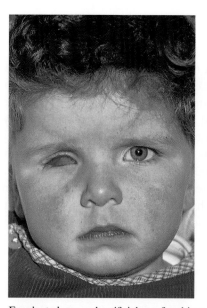
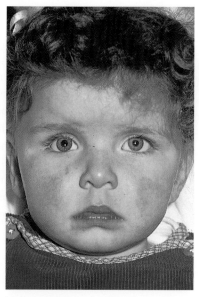

Enucleated eye and artificial eye fitted in a child treated for retinoblastoma.

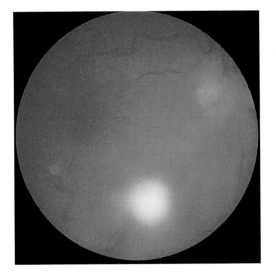

Toxocariasis. Vitreous inflammation obscures the retina around the white mass—the parasite is within this lesion.

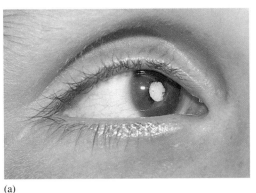

(a)

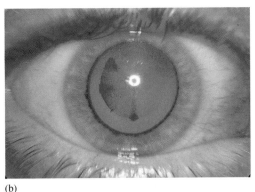

(b)

White fundus reflex—(a) complete and (b) partial (lamellar) cataract silhouetted against the red reflex.

for example galactosaemia, hypoparathyroidism or diabetes mellitis. Complete bilateral cataracts require surgical extraction as soon as the diagnosis is made, and visual rehabilitation with glasses or contact lenses prevents amblyopia from stimulus deprivation. Surgery for unilateral cataract carries a poorer outlook for central vision. Glasses cannot be worn as the large disparity between the lens power, magnification, and image size in the normal and operated eye will lead to visual confusion. A contact lens circumvents this difficulty because it is placed nearer the eye than a spectacle lens, and the magnification effect is reduced. However, contact lens fitting and occlusion of the other eye (to reverse amblyopia) does not yield good visual results as children enjoy removing contact lenses, and often lose them, seriously jeopardizing visual rehabilitation. Intraocular lens implantation in young children can lead to a severe inflammatory response, in contrast to the quieter tolerance of an implant in the adult eye. Uncertainties concerning the long-term effects of implanted intraocular lenses, and difficulties in deciding which lens power is appropriate for a growing eye, have precluded their use in children. Epikeratophakia is a technique involving a 'living contact lens' prepared from donor cornea which is sutured to the infant's aphakic cornea.

Retinopathy of prematurity

Retinopathy of prematurity (ROP) refers to all retinal changes seen in low birth weight premature babies, ranging from mild peripheral vascular arrest to advanced retinal scarring and shrinkage. Mild retinal scarring retinopathy of prematurity can lead to severe myopia, amblyopia, and squint. Progression to severe scarring disease is not common but is blinding, and prevention of late stage ROP by screening and treatment with cryotherapy or laser is now performed in most neonatal intensive care units.

Other causes of leukocoria include persistent hyperplastic primary vitreous (Part 1) and Coats' disease in which exudate leaks into the retina from abnormal bood vessels.

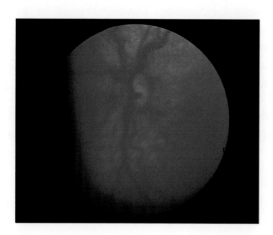

Acute retinopathy of prematurity. Dilated, tortuous retinal blood vessels seen through vitreous haze. Cryotherapy treatment is urgently required to prevent scarring disease.

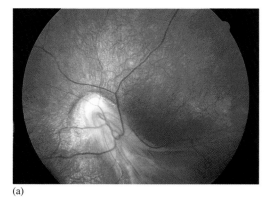

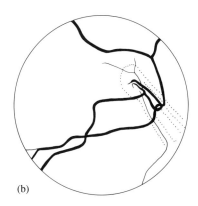

(a)

(b)

(a) Cicatricial retinopathy of prematurity. Fibrotic scarring distorts the retina and produces disc dragging.
(b) The dotted lines indicate scarred retina which distorts and drags the retinal blood vessels away from their usual course.

Inherited retinal disease

Retinitis pigmentosa

Poor night vision may be a sign of retinitis pigmentosa which may be inherited as an autosomal recessive, dominant, or X-linked trait. An adolescent complaining of poor vision in dim illumination should be suspected of suffering from retinitis pigmentosa, and the diagnosis should be confirmed by retinal examination. In the early stage of the disease clumps of pigment are seen in the peripheral retina and these slowly and progressively destroy the peripheral field, leaving only a small central island of vision in later life. There is no cure (Part 7).

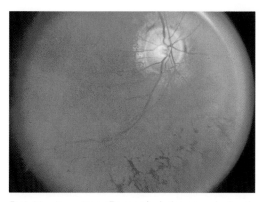

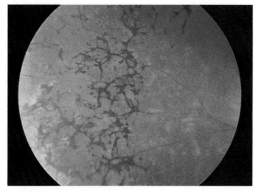

Retinitis pigmentosa. 'Bone spicules' progressively advance towards the central retina.

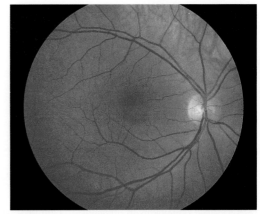

Normal macula.

Hereditary macular dystrophy. The diagnosis is made
on clinical appearance and electrophysiological
testing. (a) Cone dystrophy: increased macular
pigment in a child with nystagmus, photophobia and
poor vision. (b) Best's vitelline dystrophy: the right
macula shows a circular yellow/orange lesion and
(c) mottled disturbance at the left macula.

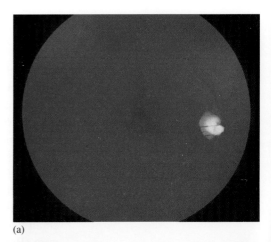

(a)

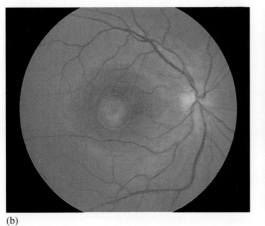

(b)

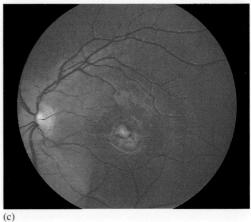

(c)

Leber's amaurosis

Leber's amaurosis is an autosomal recessive disease which affects the retinal photoreceptors early in life. Although most infants with this condition are otherwise normal, mental retardation and other neurological or renal abnormalities may be present. Children with this condition show poor pupillary light responses and may display 'paradoxical pupils' which dilate rather than constrict when stimulated by light.

Cone dystrophy

Cone dystrophy is a rare autosomal dominant disorder affecting central vision and presents with nystagmus, photophobia, and poor colour vision. An ophthalmologist can confirm the diagnosis by the clinical appearance of a 'blister' of fluid at the macula and electrophysiological testing.

Neurological disease

Visual loss due to neurological disease is often advanced on presentation and the parents may have noticed alteration in their child's visual behaviour. Observant parents may have detected abnormal eye movements, impairment of gaze, and even pupillary abnormalities. A young child is unlikely to complain of a visual field defect, though the older child with bitemporal hemianopia may complain of blurred vision or objects appearing and suddenly disappearing from view. Headache is a sign of neurological disease though can be difficult to distinguish from 'psychogenic' headache. If a headache affects a young child, is acute in onset and severe enough to alter the child's normal activities it is likely to have an organic cause. The additional features of neck stiffness and photophobia point to meningeal irritation. Raised intracranial pressure may cause nausea, vomiting, unexplained behaviour changes, and diplopia if the child has an associated VI nerve palsy (see part 4). Papilloedema caused by raised intracranial pressure does not classically produce visual symptoms, though transient dimness or visual 'blackouts' are described by some children.

Recognition of eye signs during neurological evaluation can save both sight and life. An assessment of
visual acuity, the pupils and their reactions to light, eye
movements, visual field, and ophthalmoscopy may lead
to the detection of a craniopharyngioma, chiasmal
glioma, or a blocked shunt.

The pupils

Unequal pupil sizes (anisocoria), for example one enlarged pupil, may be due to instillation of dilating drops
or, more seriously, a III nerve palsy (see part 4). Adie's
pupil is also a cause of a large pupil which reacts poorly
to light. The cause of this seemingly benign condition is
not known. A small irregularly shaped pupil could indicate uveitis (Part 7), and a small circular pupil may be a
sign of Horner's syndrome. This results from sympathetic
denervation to the eye and the structures affected are
the pupil, lids, and sweat glands producing the clinical
triad of meiosis (small pupil), ptosis, and anhydrosis.
The sympathetic supply may be interrupted anywhere
between the superior cervical ganglion and the eye,
therefore possible causes include birth trauma or cardio-
thoracic surgery. The remote possibility of a tumour
should be excluded by chest X-ray, and head and neck
CT imaging. Children with congenital Horner's syndrome may have impaired iris pigmentation leading to
different coloured irides (heterochromia). Heterochromia is also sometimes found in children with
uveitis.

Pupillary light reactions

When a bright torch light shines into the eye, the pupil
briskly constricts in both eyes and in the dark, both
dilate. The direct light test shows the response of the
pupil in the illuminated eye, and a consensual reaction
is seen in the other eye. Attempts should be made to
encourage the child to look at a distant object and
not at the torchlight, as accommodation induces pupil
constriction. Healthy direct and consensual reactions
suggests that the optic nerve (afferent) and neural connections with the third cranial nerve (efferent) are intact. The swinging light test compares the direct and
consensual response between the two eyes. A bright

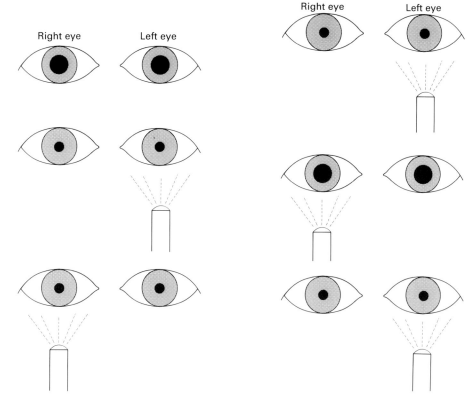

Normal pupillary light reflexes. Light shone into one eye causes pupil constriction in the same eye (direct response) and the other eye (consensual response).

The swinging light test. Impaired direct and consensual responses causes pupil dilation in both eyes as the light swings from the left to the right eye. This indicates a right afferent pupillary defect (Marcus Gunn pupil).

light is shone in one eye and then the other, whilst observing the pupil reaction in each, and this procedure is repeated several times. If one pupil dilates when the light has swung over from the other eye, it indicates a relative afferent defect and suggests retina or optic nerve dysfunction.

An apparently blind infant with no eye abnormality and normally reacting pupils may have occipital cortical damage, commonly due to birth asphyxia. Associated features include cerebral palsy, mental retardation, microcephaly, and seizures.

Visual field testing

The normal field of vision is the shape of a pear lying on its side, with the stalk pointing inwards, and the broad base extending out. The pointed parts of the 'pear' for each eye lie on the bridge of the nose, where right and left fields overlap. Gross visual field defects may be detected by adapting the confrontation test to the child's age and ability. The examiner holds the attention of the child with a pentorch light or toy, while a second toy is introduced from the periphery which, if seen, causes the child to turn towards it. More accurate testing is possible in older children by asking the patient to fix their gaze straight ahead (on to the examiner's eye) and to cover the other eye. Targets are introduced into the peripheral field in all quadrants and the child is asked 'When can you see the toy out of the corner of your eye?'. Tumours causing chiasmal compression, for example craniopharyngioma, damage crossing nerve fibres causing bitemporal hemianopia, which is often far advanced before detection. Homonymous field defects affect the same section of visual field in both eyes and result from lesions in the higher visual pathway and cerebral cortex.

Gaze palsy

Disorders of vertical gaze occur in hydrocephalus. The eye appearance is called the 'setting sun' sign and is often accompanied by visual loss, though this usually resolves following shunt surgery. Horizontal gaze palsies may develop in patients with Arnold–Chiari malformation, and certain metabolic disorders, for example maple syrup urine disease.

Papilloedema and optic atrophy

Examination of the optic nerve head in a child is not easy, so one must look for other clues such as defective pupillary responses to light, a poor visual acuity, or impaired visual field. Although these signs are present in a child with post-viral optic neuritis, they are likely to be normal if the swollen nerve heads are the result of raised intracranial pressure, in which case hydrocephalus may be present. A swollen, oedematous nerve looks indistinct and raised in comparison to the normal optic nerve. Formerly, the optic nerve was termed the papilla, so the term papilloedema was coined. The diagnosis can be difficult to make—conditions which closely

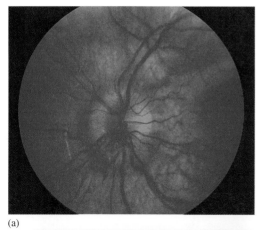

(a)

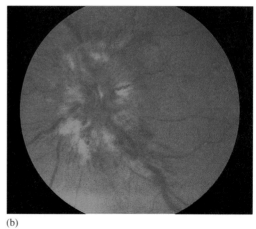

(b)

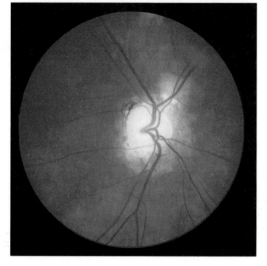

(c)

Papilloedema at early (a) established (b) and advanced (c) stages.

Optic atrophy.

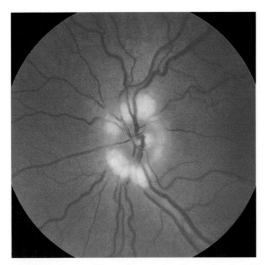

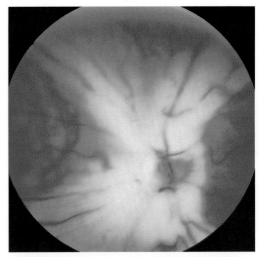

Myelinated nerve fibres obscure the disc and retinal blood vessels and can mimic disc swelling. Retinal nerve fibres are normally non-myelinated.

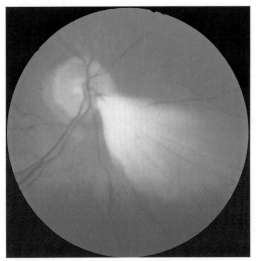

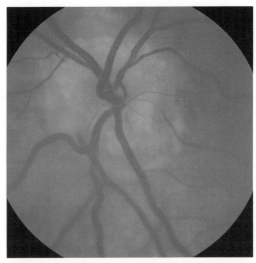

Myelinated nerve fibres delineate the arcuate pattern of retinal nerve fibres. This is a benign condition and the vision is unaffected.

Optic nerve head drusen: hyaline deposits buried within the disc can mimic disc swelling

mimic papilloedema include hypermetropic discs, myelinated nerve fibres, and hyaline bodies (drusen), a congenital anomaly of the optic disc. Chronic papilloedema leads to optic atrophy and visual loss, and when this has occurred the nerve cannot become swollen again despite raised intracranial pressure. If a child with a ventriculo-peritoneal shunt has optic atrophy and progressively deteriorating vision, a blocked shunt should be suspected.

The parents may have noticed associated nystagmus or squint and even comment on abnormal pupil reactions of a child with optic atrophy. The diagnosis is further suspected by poor pupillary light responses and pallor of the optic nerve head. Other causes of optic atrophy are perinatal anoxia, chiasmal compression, trauma, and meningitis. Optic atrophy may be inherited as an autosomal dominant or recessive trait. Metabolic disorders associated with optic atrophy include diabetes insipidus and mellitis. A diagnosis of optic atrophy is made difficult in the infant because of the normally pale appearance of the disc, therefore an ophthalmic referral is necessary. Electrodiagnostic tests help to make the diagnosis. The visual outlook for children with optic atrophy may be unpredictable and late improvement may occur particularly when associated with meningoencephalitis or hydrocephalus.

Nystagmus

The term nystagmus refers to rhythmic involuntary movements of the eyes which may be a sign of neurological disease. The nystagmus may have horizontal and vertical components, be pendular, with oscillations of the eyes of equal speed in each direction, or jerking, with a fast movement in one direction followed by a slower recovery movement in the opposite direction. Unusual vertical forms of acquired nystagmus occur in a number of neurological diseases affecting the visual pathways, and particularly the optic chiasm. While individually rare, these diseases are very significant as they include optic nerve glioma, craniopharyngioma and other tumours. Diseases of the cerebellum, vestibular connections, midbrain, and cerebral hemispheres may also cause nystagmus. A child with albinism, inherited retinal disease, and optic disc abnormalities may have nystagmus.

If investigation fails to reveal an underlying neurological or ocular disease the child is likely to have primary congenital nystagmus. This first becomes apparent within the first three months of life. The key characteristic is that the nystagmus is jerking, and only occurs in a horizontal direction. The nystagmus remains comitant, and horizontal in all directions of gaze. Sometimes the nystagmus has a much lower amplitude when the child looks to one side and this may lead to a compensatory head posture with the head turned towards the opposite side. Hypermetropic astigmatism is often present and should be corrected optically. Contact lens correction may be more effective than spectacle correction, particularly in teenagers. Near vision is usually good enough to allow mainstream education.

Roving eye movements are observed in children with profound visual loss. The fixation reflexes develop within the first three to four months of life, during which time the normal child may exhibit uncoordinated eye movements. Persistence of abnormal eye movements after this age raises the possibility of profound visual deprivation. The eyes wander as if they are attempting to fix, producing a characteristic 'searching' nystagmus. The movements are relatively slow and normally some underlying cause such as congenital cataracts, Leber's congenital amaurosis, cicatricial retinopathy of prematurity, or cortical blindness is evident on further examination.

If there is a suspicion of nystagmus, gaze palsy, papilloedema, or optic atrophy the child must be investigated urgently by a paediatric neurologist and an ophthalmologist.

PART FOUR

Squint

Squint

The age at which strabismus is detected is determined by the nature of the squint, the powers of observation of other family members, and the success of primary care screening. A squint may be constant and present all the time. If it is noticed only when the child is tired it is called a latent squint. The onset of concomitant convergent strabismus may coincide with a period of illness, for example whooping cough or chickenpox. A child with a divergent squint may complain of eyestrain and headache when reading, and have a tendency to close one eye in bright sunshine though the reason for this is unclear. Questions which should be asked during the history taking are: Who first suspected a squint and when? What is the duration, severity, and progression of the squint? Can the child see toys, books, television, and the blackboard? How is the child developing physically and intellectually? Was the birth normal? Is there a family history of squint?

Examination

First of all the examiner should assess the visual acuity as parents are unlikely to be aware of the presence of subnormal vision in one eye. The presence of a squint is assessed by examining the corneal light reflexes, testing the eye movements, and performing the cover test.

Corneal light reflexes

The corneal light reflex test provides an assessment of ocular alignment, and is performed by holding a pentorch one metre from the child, and observing the reflections of the beam from the cornea. These reflections should be slightly nasal to the corneal centre (in the central pupillary area) if the visual axes are parallel. If one light reflex falls more nasal to this position a divergent appearance is noted, and if temporally located, a convergent appearance is seen. Prominent epicanthal

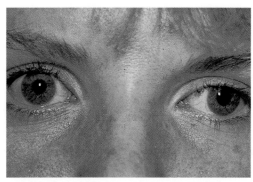

Left divergent squint. The light reflex is displaced nasal to the left pupil.

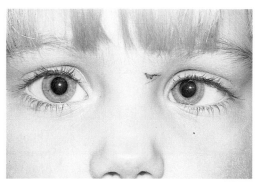

Left convergent squint. The light reflex is displaced temporal to the left pupil.

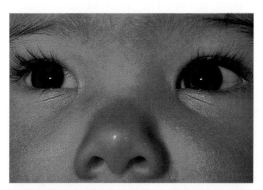

Medial epicanthal folds partially occluding the nasal sclera, giving the impression of a convergent squint.

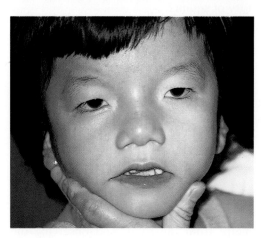

Hypertelorism. Widely spaced eyes may give the impression of a divergent squint.

folds can mimic a convergent squint; it is helpful to pinch the bridge of the nose gently exposing the hidden sclera. This manoeuvre will improve the appearance of the apparent squint. A wider than normal space between the two eyes is called 'hypertelorism', and this can mimic a divergent squint.

Eye movements

Examination of eye movements for restriction or over-action of motility in all positions of gaze, is the next step. Testing ocular motility in an infant can be crudely assessed by holding and turning the baby. As the infant fixes his gaze upon the examiner's face, one may observe the horizontal eye movements as the infant is moved from side to side, and the vertical movements as he is tipped back and forth. An older child with good visual acuity is able to hold fixation on a small toy and this makes it possible to test the nine cardinal positions of gaze. The examiner should get down to the child's level and hold a target upon which the child can fix his gaze. This can be a pentorch for an infant or a small toy or picture in an older child. With the child looking straight ahead (primary position) and without moving the target, the position of the lids, pupils, and corneal light reflexes should be observed. Next, the target is moved to the left, right, up, and then down, whilst watching for inability of either eye to move fully in any of these directions. Eye motility in the remaining positions of gaze may now be tested—up and right, down and right, up and left, down and left positions. If one eye does not appear to achieve one extreme of gaze, a cover/uncover test can substantiate the suspicion, and this is described below. Often the child moves his head to follow the target and may violently resent attempts at head restraint. This problem is overcome by allowing the child to turn his head and to take the target past the point of maximum head turn.

Cover/uncover test

This test helps to detect a manifest squint. This test should be done at the child's eye level and using an appropriate fixation target the child's eyes are held in the primary position of gaze. Then one eye is covered whilst watching for movement in the uncovered eye in taking up fixation of the target. Covering the eye of an infant with the examiner's thumb is less threatening than a plastic or card occluder. Moving the target and watching for corresponding movement ensures the eye is fixed and looking at the object. When the left eye is covered, if the right eye turns out to fix on the target

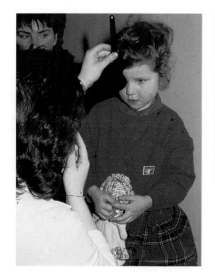

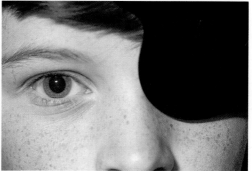

Cover test.

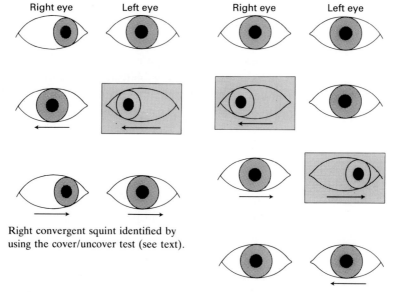

Right convergent squint identified by
using the cover/uncover test (see text).

Latent divergent strabismus identified by
using the alternating cover test (see text).

there is a right convergent squint. If the right eye turns
in to fix on the target there is a right divergent squint. If
the right eye fixes on and follows the target there is no
squint in the right eye. However, if the right eye does
not move to follow the target the child cannot see the

target with this eye. Next, the eye is uncovered and the examiner watches for a return movement of the eyes. This return movement will not be observed in a child who is able to fix well with either eye; however, the strabismic child who preferentially fixes with the uncovered eye will show a return movement. The procedure may be repeated to confirm any deviation or refixation movements of either eye and when the findings have been recorded, the cover/uncover test is performed on the other eye. The figure on page 64 illustrates the cover test in a child with a right convergent squint.

A concomitant convergent squint presents early in life, and is associated with amblyopia and hypermetropia. The sooner occlusion treatment is started, the better is the visual result.

A latent squint is present in many children and is a tendency for an eye to drift into a convergent or divergent position but is controlled through the stimulus of maintaining binocular single vision. If a child is tired or unwell, control of the latent squint may be undermined and a manifest squint can be unmasked temporarily or permanently. The convergence insufficiency associated with latent divergence may produce the symptoms of eyestrain and headache when reading, or diplopia. The alternating cover test is performed to detect a latent squint. The examiner begins as if performing a cover/ uncover test with the child looking at a target in the primary position. One eye is covered, and by moving the target and observing the eye following, fixation is confirmed. Next, instead of taking the cover away altogether, the cover is swiftly switched to the opposite eye. Repeatedly switching the cover from one eye to the other prevents the binocular clues needed to control a latent squint, and it becomes unmasked. A refixation movement of the covered eye as it is uncovered can be interpreted using the same guide outlined above.

Children with a latent divergent squint are often myopic, and with time the squint may become constant. If by this stage binocular vision is well established, the risk of amblyopia is reduced.

Profound visual loss in one eye of an older child will often result in a divergent squint; while the better eye is used the other eye drifts into a position of constant divergence.

Treatment

A child with suspected squint must be referred to an ophthalmologist, who can confirm the diagnosis, and exclude coexisting eye disease. Contrary to popular belief, squints do not cure themselves, not all squints require surgery, and strabismic amblyopia is not only found in large angle squints but may also be present in the smallest angle squint. When a diagnosis of non-paralytic squint is made and the eyes are found to be disease-free, the priority should be to maximize the visual potential of both eyes.

Non-surgical treatment

Swift correction of refractive error and amblyopia with glasses and occlusion therapy aims to improve the visual function in some children and may improve the appearance of the squint. If occlusion therapy is successful in improving vision in a squinting amblyopic eye, the squint may then alternate between the eyes. This indicates that the child can fix with either eye— the parents may be alarmed by the apparent shift of the squint from one eye to the other eye, and they should be reassured that this alternation is the goal of occlusion therapy. It is at this stage that surgery may be considered.

Orthoptic exercises to improve convergence ability may improve control of a latent divergent squint, though if the squint becomes manifest (present constantly) and diplopia is noticed then surgery should be considered.

Surgery

When the child's visual potential has been realized using the methods described above, surgery to correct the cosmetic appearance may be considered. A squinting child starting school is often subject to a barrage of insults, therefore surgery should be performed before this time, and when the angle is large an operation may be advised before two years of age. Squint surgery is one of the most common electively performed operations in childhood, and the aim is to realign the visual axes by adjusting the length and position of the muscles on the surface of the eyeball. All procedures are carried out under general anaesthetic and usually only one eye is operated on at one sitting. If the angle of the squint is very large bilateral squint operations may be necessary. In order to correct a convergent squint, the medial rectus muscle is detached from its insertion and re-attached further back to the sclera. This has the effect of letting out or weakening the effect of the muscle (recession). The lateral rectus is shortened by excising a length and reattaching it back to the original insertion. This enhances or strengthens the action of the muscle (resection). The amount of recession and resection depends on the size of the squint. Most surgeons use absorbable sutures, precluding the need for routine removal. Usually the eye is not covered with a pad after the surgery. The child is discharged from hospital the day after surgery with an eye that is a little red and sore, but comfort quickly returns. Antibiotic ointment keeps the wounds clean and reminds both parents and child of the recent eye operation, and that it should be protected for several weeks from the chlorine of a swimming pool, and the sand from the local pit!

Early surgery may bring the return of three dimensional perception (assuming it was there to start with) though this theoretical goal is rarely achieved. In practice, a lesser form of binocular vision allows the two visual images to be fused into one (without the finer degrees of depth appreciation) which maintains the eyes in a straight ahead position.

Ocular muscle palsy

This results from direct or indirect damage to the cranial nerves III, IV, and VI. An oculomotor or III nerve palsy affects the function of all the extraocular muscles apart from the lateral rectus and the superior oblique, and the eye assumes a 'down and out' position. In addition the levator muscle innervation is affected producing a ptosis, and the innervation to the pupil sphincter is impaired leading to a dilated pupil—the three cardinal signs of a III nerve palsy. The trochlear or IV nerve supplies the superior oblique muscle and the motility of the eye is impaired on looking down and

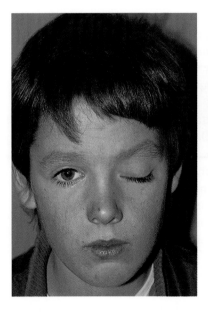

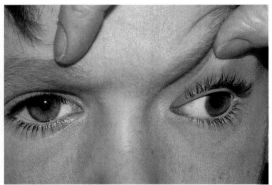

Left III (oculomotor) nerve palsy. Ptosis, the eye is 'down and out' and the pupil is enlarged.

in towards the nose. The abducens or VI nerve supplies the lateral rectus, and a palsy would weaken lateral eye movement and cause an incomitant convergent squint (Part 2). A young child is able to suppress the image from the deviating eye in order to avoid visual confusion, but the older child cannot and will notice double vision or diplopia. If the diplopia is long-standing he will have a compensatory head posture as an adaptive measure to minimize this diplopia. The angle of the paralytic squint will be largest in the direction in which the paralysed muscle would normally act, for example with a left lateral rectus palsy the squint angle would be greatest on left gaze but in other directions the visual axes are aligned. Incomitant strabismus may also be associated with congenital syndromes, for example Duane's retraction syndrome which is caused by abnormal innervation of the medial and lateral recti muscles. When the child attempts to look to one side there is limitation of abduction with widening of the palpebral fissure. On looking to the opposite side, adduction is mildly impaired and there is narrowing of the palpebral fissure. Another example of a squint syndrome is Brown's superior oblique tendon sheath syndrome which causes restriction of this muscle and the eye fails to elevate in the adducted position. Although these

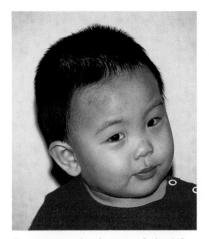

Compensatory head posture facing left with chin down. This boy has a right superior oblique paresis, and adopts this head posture to avoid diplopia.

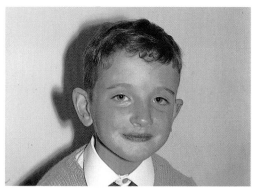 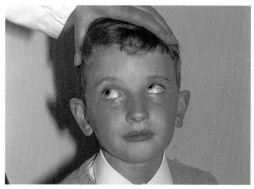

The left superior oblique is paretic, and the subsequent overaction of the inferior oblique causes the left eye to overshoot upwards.

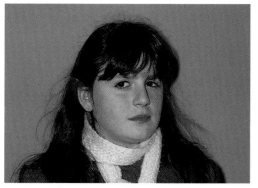 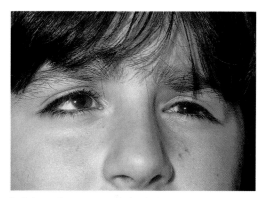

Compensatory head posture facing to the left. This girl has a lateral rectus paresis, and by facing towards the direction of the paretic muscle she avoids diplopia.

Left lateral rectus paresis is obvious on left gaze.

syndromes are non-progressive, amblyopia should be treated; eye muscle surgery may also be required to realign the eyes and rectify the compensatory head posture.

Intracranial disease should be suspected if a child acquires a paralytic squint.

PART FIVE

Watering eye

Red eye

Trauma

Watering eye

Nasolacrimal duct obstruction

The nasolacrimal duct drains tears and microscopic debris from the lacrimal sac to the nose. 1–2 per cent of infants have delayed patency of their nasolacrimal ducts which is usually unilateral and resolves by 9–12 months. Pooling of tears with overflow suggests nasolacrimal duct blockage, and predisposes the child to

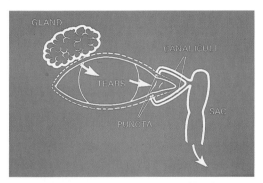

The lacrimal apparatus. Tears produced by the lacrimal gland drain into the inferior meatus of the nose via the puncti, canaliculi, lacrimal sac, and nasolacrimal duct.

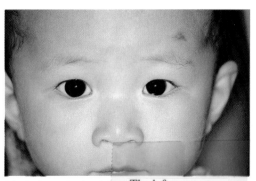

Blocked nasolacrimal duct. The left eye waters with discharge due to congenital incomplete patency of the nasolacrimal duct.

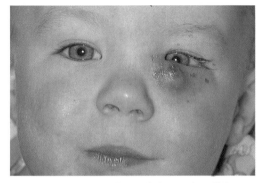

Acute dacryocystitis. Abscess below and medial to the inner canthus.

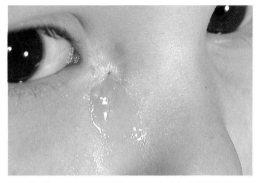

Fistula due to inappropriate surgical incision. Tears and mucopurulent discharge drain from the lacrimal sac.

recurrent bouts of mucopurulent conjunctivitis. This should be treated with lid cleansing and topical antibiotic drops. Regular massage over the lacrimal sac helps to encourage patency by breaking down membranous obstructions. Although not always successful, this simple manoeuvre can produce good results if the mother is diligent in performing the massage. Should the symptoms of watering and recurrent conjunctivitis persist after one year of age, irrigation and probing of the nasolacrimal duct under general anaesthesia is indicated. An acute dacryocystitis results from infection and distension of the lacrimal sac, due to a blockage of the nasolacrimal duct. Antibiotics control the infection and probing the nasolacrimal duct under general anaesthetic usually relieves the condition in these infants. A child with nasolacrimal duct blockage, need not be referred to an ophthalmologist unless it persists until late infancy or an acute dacryocystitis supervenes.

Glaucoma

Glaucoma is a condition of raised intraocular pressure caused by impaired drainage of aqueous humour from the eye. A child with glaucoma has tearing and photophobia exhibiting intolerance to bright lights, often by hiding their face in the blankets. The raised pressure expands the child's eyes and the corneas become progressively enlarged and cloudy. It is the pressure effects on the nerve tissue of the optic nerve together with the splits, swelling, and later scarring of the cornea which blind the child. The child should be sent immediately to the ophthalmologist for evaluation. The definitive treatment is surgical, though topical antiglaucoma medication and systemic acetazolamide reduces the intraocular pressure until surgery is performed.

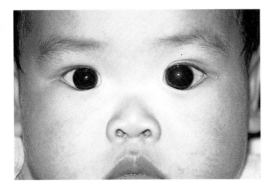

Buphthalmos. The corneal diameter of the left eye is enlarged.

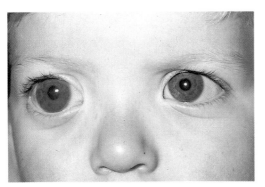

Buphthalmos. Both corneal diameters are enlarged.

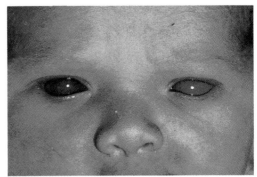

The blue/green haze suggests oedema within the cornea.

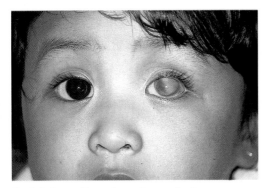

Buphthalmos. Corneal scarring results from prolonged oedema.

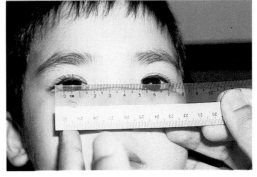

Measuring the corneal diameter. The distance from the nasal to temporal iris border should be less than 12.0 mm and equal in both eyes.

Red eye

A constellation of eye diseases can present as a red eye. The key in discriminating between the trivial and self limiting and the serious, is the attention to coexisting signs. Good observation and confidence in interpreting these signs will lead to a diagnosis.

Infection

Ophthalmia neonatorum

An infant less than 30 days of age with a severe muco-purulent conjunctivitis has ophthalmia neonatorum. The lids are oedematous and swollen and the cornea should be examined for signs of ulceration for it is this which can lead to blindness.

All children suspected of suffering from such an infection need urgent referral to an ophthalmology/paediatric team, as certain pathogens, gonococcus in particular, can melt away the cornea and enter the eye within 24 hours. Chlamydial ophthalmia, transmitted by maternal genital contact may be associated with otitis and pneumonitis and requires systemic antibiotic treatment.

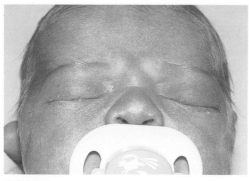

Ophthalmia neonatorum.

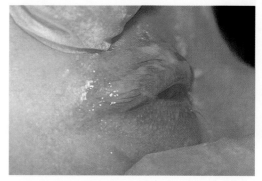

Swollen, sticky lids maybe difficult to prise apart and bathing the lid margins may ease opening. Take care—high pressure pus may produce a jet!

Bacterial conjunctivitis

A baby with a recurrent sticky and watering eye may have a blocked nasolacrimal duct (see page 73). Infection (when the duct is patent) settles quickly with topical antibiotic drops instilled 2 hourly for the first 2 days, then 4 hourly for 5 days.

Viral conjunctivitis

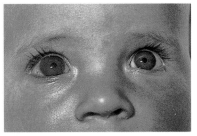

This presents with redness and watering and accompanies an upper respiratory tract infection. Preauricular lymphadenopathy may be present. Resolution should occur within two weeks. Lid cleansing and topical antibiotic drops prevent a secondary bacterial infection and good hygiene should be practised to prevent spread to other family members.

Viral conjunctivitis. A red and watering eye with no mucopus.

Toxoplasmosis

Active toxoplasmosis retinitis may present as a red eye and is due to maternal ingestion of undercooked meat or exposure to cat or dog faeces. Inflammation in the anterior chamber, vitreous, and retina cause poor vision, and obscure the red reflex and retinal detail during ophthalmoscopy.

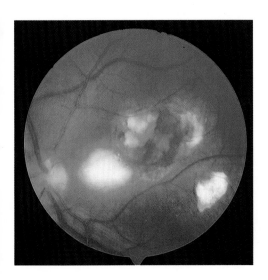

Toxoplasmosis. A reactivated focus of infection adjacent to the optic nerve appears white and fluffy—a hyperpigmented scar indicates past infection.

Allergy

Hay fever associated conjunctivitis

Itchy red eyes in atopic children (with asthma, eczema, or hay fever) and the presence of a stringy mucoid discharge with an itch/rub cycle suggest an allergic aetiology. Avoiding the allergen if possible and using topical sodium cromoglycate drops four times daily, helps this condition.

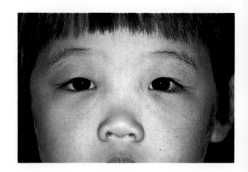

Hay fever conjunctivitis. Irritable, swollen lids and conjunctiva.

Vernal keratoconjunctivitis

This allergic disease can produce severe and debilitating corneal damage. These children should be managed by an ophthalmologist. Pain, photophobia, and watering are intense and the large corneal ulcers can scar and permanently impair vision. Treatment includes the use of sodium cromoglycate drops, which prevent mast cell degranulation by stabilizing the cell membranes, and reducing the intense inflammatory reaction with topical steroids.

Remember that steroids can encourage infection and lead to cataract and glaucoma.

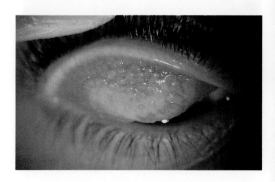

Vernal disease. Flat-topped papillae beneath upper lid—mild disease.

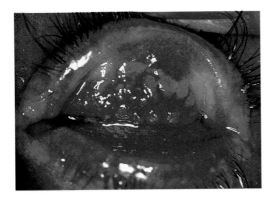

Vernal disease. Profuse watering and redness—acute and severe exacerbation.

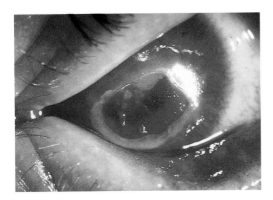

Corneal ulcer associated with vernal disease stained at the ulcer edge with Rose Bengal dye.

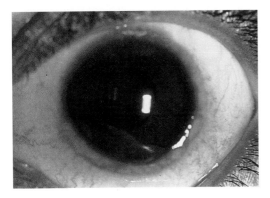

Limbal vernal disease. Swelling around the limbus in an Indian child.

Corneal epithelial disease can lead to infected corneal ulceration

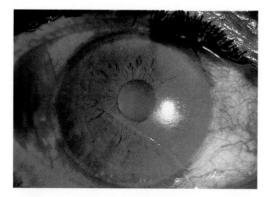

Disrupted corneal light reflex. Dry unhealthy epithelium produces a lacklustre appearance.

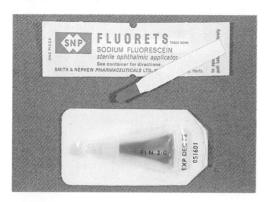

Fluorescein is available as a 2% solution, or impregnated into a dry paper strip to be wetted before use.

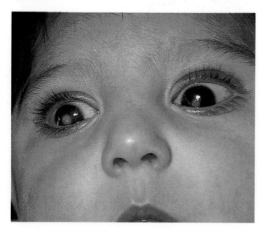

Fluorescein stains the abraded surface and looks green.

Bacterial corneal ulcer

Predisposing factors include malnutrition (vitamin A deficiency), debilitating infections (measles), and neglected trauma (corneal foreign body, abrasion). A milky white fluid level in the anterior chamber suggests pus (hypopyon) and intraocular spread of the infection.

Infected corneal ulcer.

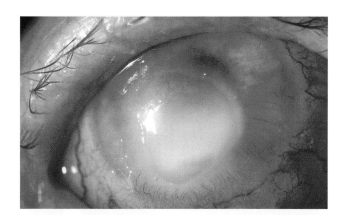

Bacterial ulcer. Anterior illumination slit shows discontinuity of the ulcerated surface.

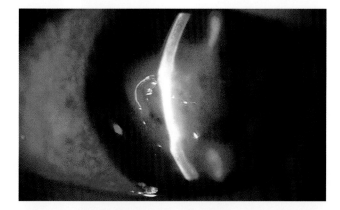

Hypopyon filling half of the anterior chamber.

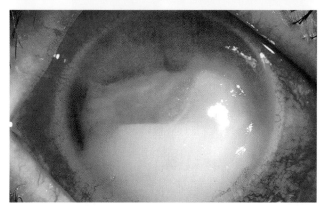

Viral corneal ulcer

Herpes simplex infection of the cornea produces a characteristic branching or dendritic ulcer which is easily identified with the help of fluorescein, which stains and highlights the denuded corneal surface. The child may also have a coldsore on the lip or a vesicular blepharitis. If a herpetic aetiology is suspected treatment should be acyclovir ointment five times a day and referral to an eye department is recommended. Inappropriate steroid treatment encourages viral replication causing overwhelming corneal destruction and blindness.

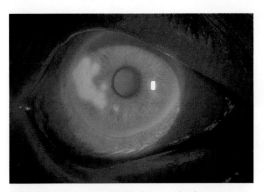

Dendritic ulcer stained with fluorescein dye.

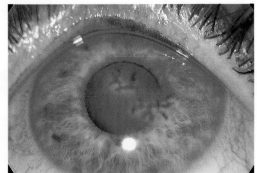

Dendritic ulcer stained with fluorescein and Rose Bengal dyes.

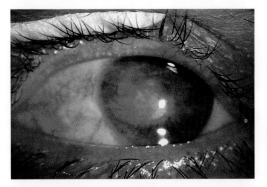

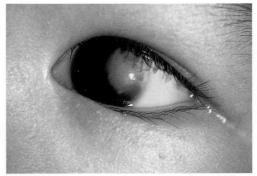

Vascularized cornea following herpetic corneal infection, leads to a dense white scar after several years.

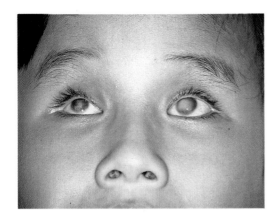

Bilateral corneal opacity following measles.

Trauma

Ocular injury is an important cause of visual handicap in childhood. The variety is wide from blunt trauma with stones (thrown or catapulted) to penetrating injury with a bow and arrow, or air gun pellet. It is important to be on the alert for the unexplained accident in the young child which may be due to violence within the home, the so-called 'battered baby' syndrome.

Periorbital bruising

The lids and orbit are good protectors of the eyeball. A black eye is the result of bleeding in and around the eyelids and is a common cause of ptosis. The lid should always be lifted to check that the eyeball is healthy and that the eye movements are full.

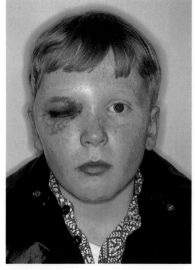

Periorbital bruising. A 'black eye' with ptosis.

Subconjunctival haemorrhage

The trauma associated with normal or forceps-assisted delivery, or severe coughing bout in a child with whooping cough can cause a rupture of small blood vessels and produce a subconjunctival haemorrhage which resolves without local treatment.

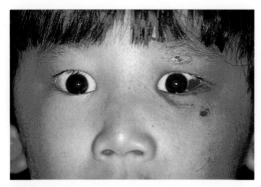

Subconjunctival haemorrhage involving temporal aspect of conjunctiva.

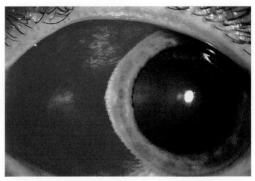

Subconjunctival haemorrhage completely obscures the conjunctival blood vessel pattern.

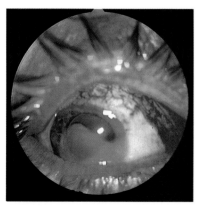

Lime burn of cornea and conjunctiva
stained with fluorescein.

Chemical injury

Disinfectants, detergents, paints, glues, and perfumes
splashed into the eye should be irrigated immediately
with clean tap water by washing with clean hands. Most
chemicals found in the home are harmless, though
strong bleach and detergents can burn the lid margin,
conjunctival and corneal surface and later scar. Children whose eyes have been in contact with these sub-
stances need urgent ophthalmological evaluation and
treatment.

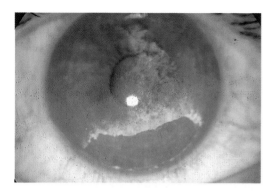

Calcified corneal opacity following lime burn.

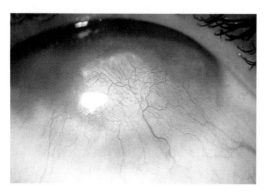

Vascularization of the cornea after chemical injury.

Lid laceration

Cuts of the eyelids, if superficial and clean can be
treated conservatively, but full thickness dirty wounds,
for instance dog bite injuries which commonly affect
the medial canthal region require cleansing, careful
examination, and repair under general anaesthetic.

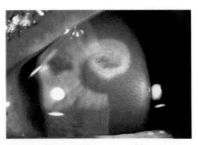

Circular corneal ulcer caused by a fingernail injury.

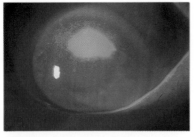

Corneal abrasion stained with fluorescein. Epithelial cells from the ulcer margin will invade to cover and heal the defect.

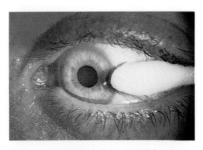

Removing a superficial corneal foreign body after instilling topical anaesthetic.

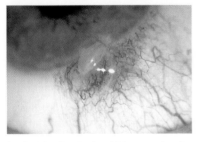

Limbal foreign body which proved to be bird seed!

Corneal abrasion

This can easily be diagnosed with fluorescein which stains the abraded epithelial area. Antibiotic ointment, a mydriatic, and a pad aid rapid healing.

Subtarsal foreign body

This diagnosis may be suggested by a history of exposure to dust or sand on a beach visit for example. The eye is red and very painful, and following instillation of fluorescein 2 per cent dye, or a fluorescein impregnated paper strip, an 'ice rink' pattern of epithelial scratches is seen on the superior cornea. Eversion of the lid is a simple procedure, and removal of the foreign body brings instant relief. The upper lid lashes are grasped and the child asked to look down. A blunt glass rod is then pressed into the upper lid skin and the lid everted, holding the lid in this position with the examiner's thumb against the lashes. A clean moistened cotton tipped bud can then be used to gently wipe away the foreign body. Releasing the lid and getting the child to look up, returns the lid to its normal position. No other treatment is required unless there is a breach of the corneal surface as seen by an area of fluorescein staining in which case topical antibiotic ointment allows healing by lubricating the eyelid/corneal interface and prevents infection of the traumatized surface.

Corneal foreign body

Any foreign body can embed itself into the corneal epithelium and produce redness surrounding the cornea. If superficial, the foreign body can be lifted off after instilling topical local anaesthetic drops and using a cotton tipped bud, or a needle. Metallic particles which become more deeply embedded may erode into the stroma and leave a 'rust ring' while the surrounding corneal tissue forms a scar. The rust remnant is best removed by an ophthalmologist, who can view the cornea through a microscope or slit lamp and safely remove deeply embedded material. In the very young or uncooperative child a short general anaesthetic allows safe removal.

Hyphaema

Blunt trauma to the eye or penetrating injuries cause intraocular bleeding, appearing as a red fluid level in the anterior chamber—a hyphaema. An unreactive semidilated pupil—traumatic mydriasis—is often present, but this requires no specific treatment. Admission to hospital for rest and observation is advisable, though it is difficult to restrain a healthy child from boisterous activities for any period of time! With rest, the hyphaema often completely absorbs within a few days; however, occasionally even a small bleed may be followed some hours or days later by a haemorrhage of much greater severity. This can be catastrophic, as the consequent intraocular pressure rise forces blood into the cornea, leaving a permanent pigment stain. Surgical evacuation is therefore indicated for this rare complication.

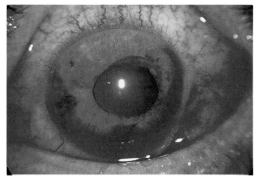

Traumatic hyphaema with mydriasis. Injury to the pupil sphincter produces an irregularly enlarged pupil.

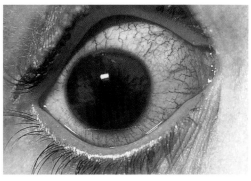

'Spontaneous' hyphaema may be caused by iris xanthogranuloma, blood dyscrasia, or non-accidental injury.

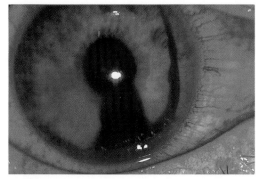

Secondary hyphaema. Rebleeding from the 12 o'clock position produced a dark clot adherent to the pupillary area reducing vision.

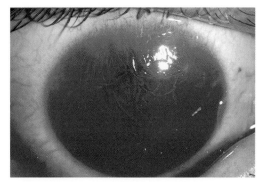

Secondary hyphaema fills the anterior chamber with raised intraocular pressure and corneal oedema (disrupting the corneal light reflex).

Vitreous, retinal, and optic nerve damage

Bleeding into the vitreous cavity and retina can occur with severe blunt trauma to the eye or rapid decelerating head injuries. In the absence of a convincing history non accidental injury or the battered baby syndrome should be suspected. Concussional injuries can cause bruising or commotio retinae, retinal breaks, and ruptures of deeper structures. Even seemingly trivial blunt injury can disrupt the blood supply to the optic nerve, which devastates the visual function and results in a pale atrophic optic nerve.

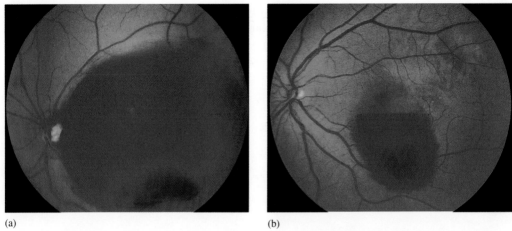

(a)   (b)

Non-accidental injury, (a) severe shaking has resulted in a large subhyaloid haemorrhage (anterior to the retina but behind the vitreous), (b) a fluid level has formed with darker blood below. Although the blood absorbs, the retinal scarring causes permanent visual loss.

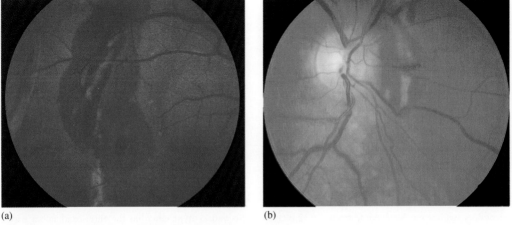

(a)   (b)

Traumatic choroidal rupture. The haemorrhagic rupture represents a break in tissue underlying the retina, resulting in a white semilunar scar months later (b).

Orbital blow out fracture

A direct blow on the eye can cause a sudden rise in intraorbital pressure and fracture the thin bone forming the orbital floor, or medial wall (into the ethmoid sinuses) with incarceration of fat or extraocular muscle. This can be the result of a tennis ball or a fist impact on to the orbit. The child will have lid bruising, double vision (if both eyes are open), a sunken eye or enophthalmos, and may exhibit crepitus with ethmoid fractures or lower lid sensation impairment if the infraorbital nerve is damaged. Referral to an ophthalmologist allows the diagnosis to be confirmed, usually with the help of a CT scan, to define the extent and site of injury. Early surgery to release entrapped tissue is usually required.

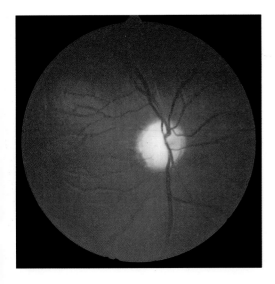

Traumatic optic atrophy. A pale nerve and profound visual loss have resulted from relatively mild trauma.

Penetrating eye injuries

Sharp projectiles of metal or glass or sharp pointed instruments such as knives, scissors, safety pins, or sharp pointed toys can perforate the cornea or sclera. Prevention is better than cure. A perforating injury may be plugged by prolapsed iris tissue producing a peaked pupil with associated hyphaema. Excessive force should not be used in prising open the lids particularly if a penetrating injury is suspected as the intraocular contents may extrude through the wound. A

general anaesthetic is needed to establish the full extent
of the injuries and to perform a primary repair of the
globe; urgent referral is always necessary.

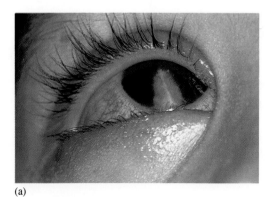

(a)

Corneal scar following a penetrating injury.

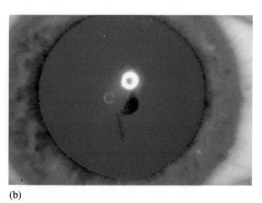

(b)

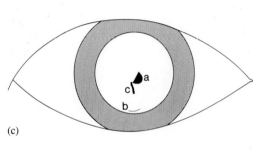

(c)

Intraocular foreign body. The metallic fragment (a) entered through a self-sealing corneal laceration (b) and
lodged in the lens through a vertical incision (c) in the lens capsule.

PART SIX

Eyelids and orbit

Eyelids and orbit

The eyelids and eyelashes are often overlooked during the eye examination but if diseased are a potent source of irritation, eye rubbing, and if left untreated can cause conjunctival and corneal problems. Allergy and infection should be diagnosed early and treated quickly to prevent these complications. Pupil occluding lid malpositions may lead to amblyopia unless swiftly treated.

Ptosis

The main muscle of upper lid elevation is the levator palpebrae, though frontalis muscle overaction may partially lift the lid to compensate for levator dysfunction. This leads to the raised eyebrow and wrinkled forehead appearance in a child with ptosis. Congenitally acquired ptosis may be associated with narrowed palpebral apertures (blepharophimosis) or aberrant innervation of other muscles (Marcus Gunn jaw winking). Acquired ptosis can result from trauma or myopathy. The upper lid should always be lifted to examine the eyeball, an obvious point which is often forgotten. The upper to lower lid distance, measured with a ruler, gives an indication of the severity of the ptosis. If the lid covers the pupil, threatening sight, surgical correction is indicated.

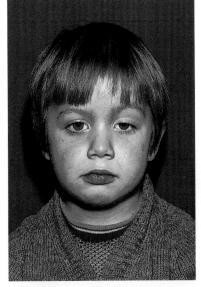

Left congenital ptosis. The visual axis remains uncovered.

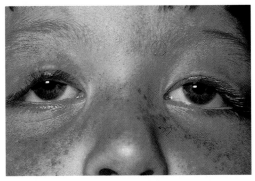

Bilateral ptosis. Symmetrical ptosis in a child with myotonic dystrophy.

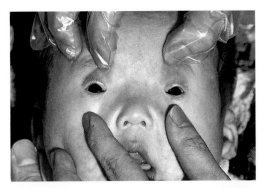

Blepharophimosis.

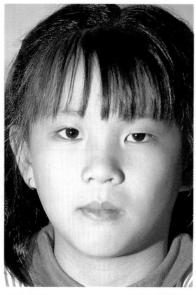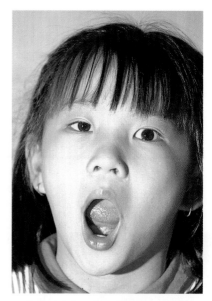

Marcus Gunn jaw winking. Left ptosis with mouth closed though the lid rises on jaw opening. This is due to abherrant neural connections between the levator muscle and the trigeminal nerve.

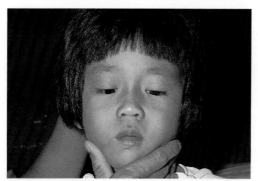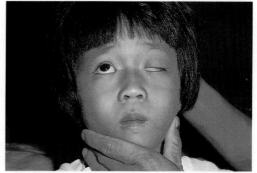

Assessing levator muscle function by observing upper lid movement from upgaze to downgaze; this child shows poor left levator function.

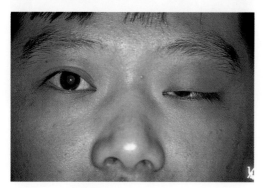

Left ptosis obscures the visual axis causing amblyopia.

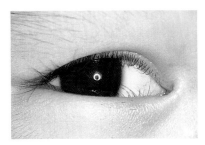

Epiblepharon with inturned lower lashes.

Epiblepharon

A prominent lower lid fold of skin inverts the lower eyelid so that the lashes rub on the cornea. This occasionally causes irritation, ulceration, and infection. If the condition does not resolve spontaneously the fold of skin can be excised surgically.

Blepharitis

This is an inflammation of the eyelids with the associated signs of itching and redness of the delicate, thin skin of the lids.

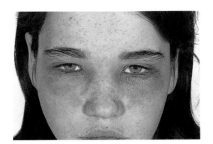

Blepharitis.

Chronic blepharitis

Crusting and discharge along the lid margin is commonly caused by a chronic staphylococcal infection which spills over on to the conjunctiva, and staphylococcal toxins can lead to corneal ulceration and scarring if left untreated.

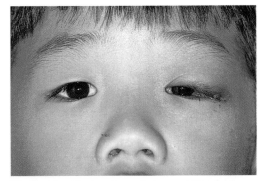

Blepharitis with chronic staphylococcal lid infection.

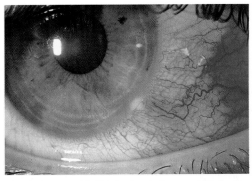

Marginal corneal infiltrate due to hypersensitivity to staphylococcal toxin.

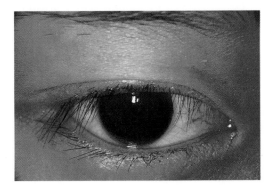

Seborrheic blepharitis showing characteristic scales and sparse lashes.

Squamous blepharitis is a chronic seborrhoeic condition with swelling, redness and scales along the eyelid margins, and loss of eyelashes; there may be an associated eczema. Bacterial colonization of the eyelids often coexists. Treatment of chronic blepharitis is to maintain the eyelid margins free of scales and crusts by lid hygiene, using cotton tipped buds and sterile saline or a 50 per cent solution of baby shampoo. The cotton tipped bud is dipped in the sterile normal saline (or cooled, freshly boiled water) and the lid margins wiped clean of scales and crusts. Topical antibiotic ointment is applied to the lid margins using a clean cotton tipped bud. This procedure is repeated two or three times a day.

Acute blepharitis

Allergic blepharitis due to local irritants such as atropine, cosmetics, nickel, and plant pollens can produce an eczematous, moist swelling of the eyelids. The offending substance should be identified and removed. If the local reaction is severe topical steroids can be used under the careful supervision of an ophthalmologist. Inappropriate and unsupervised steroid treatment can lead to blindness through steroid-related cataract and glaucoma, and encourages viral replication in a child with unsuspected herpetic eye disease.

Other causes of blepharitis

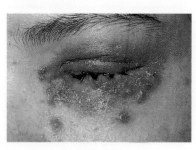

Herpes simplex blepharitis with secondary bacterial infection.

Herpes simplex blepharitis produces weeping vesicles and is treated with topical acyclovir cream. Secondary infection can be recognized by golden-yellow crusting (impetigo) and mucopurulent discharge which should be treated by lid cleansing with moist, clean cotton wool and topical antibiotic ointment. The cornea should be examined for corneal dendritic ulcers.

Pubic lice or *Pthirus pubis* can produce an intense blepharitis with itching and redness of the lids. This eyelash infestation is treated by mechanical removal of the lice and eggs. In adolescents, the pubic and axillary hair should be washed with medicated shampoo and the whole family require treatment.

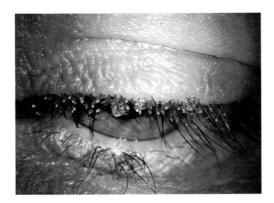

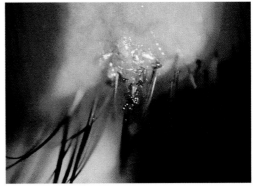

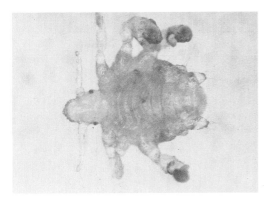

Pubic louse infestation of the lids. The nits are strongly adherent to the lashes.

Stye or hordeolum

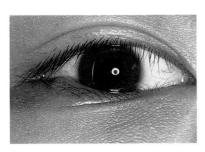

Stye.

This local infection of a superficial lash follicle requires topical antibiotic drops, and warm compresses which should lead to resolution. Otherwise the lesion will come to a head to rupture on to the skin surface.

Chalazion or meibomian cyst

These cysts often resolve or discharge spontaneously through the skin or behind the lid and require topical antibiotic drops to prevent conjunctivitis following the release of infected material. In the acute stage the child can present with a 'preseptal cellulitis' (see page 98) and is treated with hot bathing, topical and systemic antibiotics. If the cyst does not resolve spontaneously or is large enough to interfere with vision, the local ophthalmologist will incise into the lesion from the conjunctival surface and curette the contents whilst the child is under general anaesthetic.

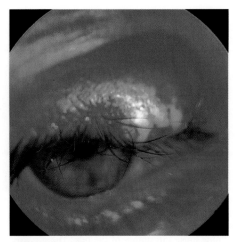

Meibomian cyst.

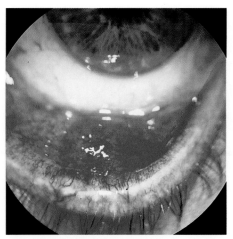

Infected meibomian cyst viewed from
the conjunctival aspect.

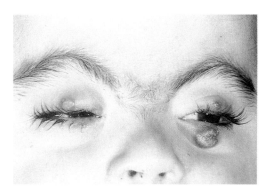

Multiple meibomian cysts in a child with DeLange
syndrome.

Preseptal and orbital cellulitis

An acute inflammation in the superficial tissues anterior
to the orbital septum is called a preseptal cellulitis or more
seriously behind it—an orbital cellulitis. A deep-seated
orbital infection can be life-threatening, spreading back-
ward to produce a cavernous sinus thrombosis and
death; therefore early diagnosis and treatment is vital.

To distinguish between a pre- and postseptal infection, the eyelids which may be red and swollen, must be
prised open to allow examination of the eyeball and
assessment of vision. If the eye can see reasonably well,
is free to move in all directions of gaze, the conjunctiva
pristine white and the pupil reactive to light, the infection
is preseptal. However, if examination shows that the
eye has poor vision, limited movement, tensely swollen

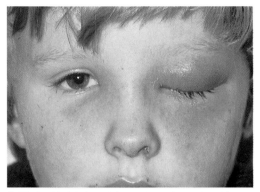

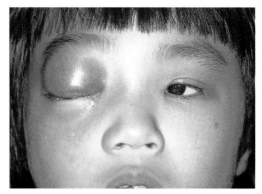

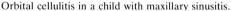

Orbital cellulitis in a child with maxillary sinusitis.

Orbital cellulitis. This child had ethmoidal sinusitis.

conjunctiva, is painfully protruding or proptosed and has a poorly reactive pupil the infection is postseptal.

Deep orbital infection may have spread from a neighbouring sinus infection, through a penetrating injury and retained foreign body, or by bloodstream carriage from a remote site of infection. The swelling behind the eye causes congestion of the retinal blood vessels, optic nerve oedema, and as already mentioned can track backwards to involve intracranial structures.

Orbital cellulitis is an alarming and life-threatening condition, best treated in hospital with systemic antibiotics and if radiological studies confirm abscess formation, urgent surgical drainage is indicated.

Molluscum contagiosum

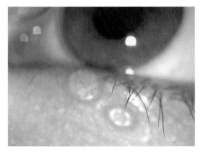

Molluscum contagiosum.

A child with a recurrently red eye may harbour a small molluscum hidden beneath the eyelashes as well as on the trunk and back. If present on the lid margin this virus shedding, umbilicated lesion causes a recurrent follicular conjunctivitis which does not improve with topical medicines. Treatment options include curettage or excision to remove the site of viral production.

Acute dacryocystitis

As discussed earlier, acute dacryocystitis is an infection of the lacrimal sac associated with a blocked nasolacrimal duct.

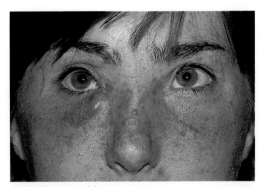

Acute dacryocystitis.

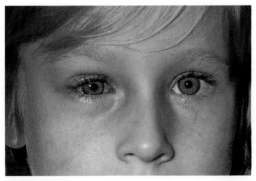

Dacryoadenitis.

Dacryoadenitis

An infection of the lacrimal gland, may have spread from a bacterial conjunctivitis or developed after a perforating injury. It can rarely complicate mumps, measles, or influenza. There is a unilateral acute, painful swelling over the upper, outer aspect of the eye, distorting the upper lid into an S shape. Systemic antibiotics are indicated if there is bacterial infection.

Dermoids

This benign developmental tumour can occur in isolation or as part of Goldenhaar's syndrome associated with preauricular skin tags. The limbal dermoid produces a cosmetic blemish and slow enlargement may distort the spherical curvature of the cornea and thereby impairs the focusing of light on the retina. Surgical excision allows the cornea to resume its normal shape, and eliminates the cosmetic blemish.

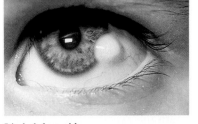

Limbal dermoid.

Orbital dermoid cyst

These inclusion, cystic lesions are usually located in the upper outer aspect of the orbit and contain sebaceous material, hair, and fat. A CT scan helps to determine the extent of the cyst, and surgical excision requires meticulous dissection.

Lid haemangioma

This may be cavernous or capillary—the former is blue in colour increasing in size when engorged with blood,

Conjunctival dermoid.

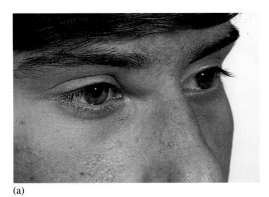

(a)

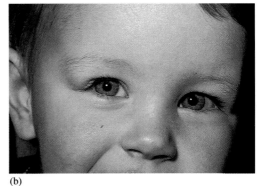

(b)

Orbital dermoid cyst sited in (a) the superomedial aspect of the orbit, (b) the superotemporal orbit.

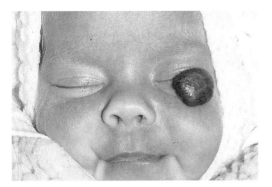

Lid haemangioma.

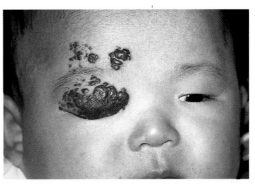

Strawberry naevus resulting in ptosis. Amblyopia will result without treatment.

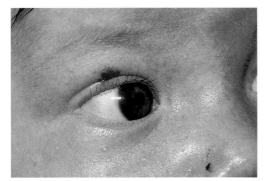

Strawberry naevus causing no threat to vision.

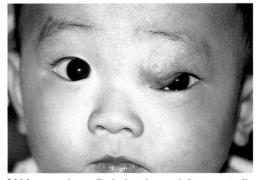

Lid haemangioma displacing the eye inferotemporally.

and the latter is a bright strawberry red. They can grow rapidly in the newborn but later spontaneously involute and diminish in size. If the pupil is covered swift intervention can avert amblyopia. The treatment options include intralesion injection of corticosteroid, laser therapy, or surgical excision.

Proptosis

The protruding eye may have an abscess or tumour sited behind the eyeball which is sight or life-threatening, and should not be missed. The differential diagnosis includes lymphangioma, haemangioma, or rhabdomyosarcoma. The appearance of proptosis may also be due to a congenitally shallow orbit associated with a cranial dysostosis. Corneal exposure can result in perforation unless protected by regular lubrication or tarsorrhaphy which involves suturing the eyelids to achieve partial closure. All children with proptosis should be promptly evaluated by an eye specialist.

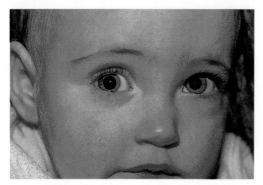
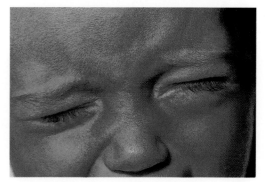

Venous varix below left eye. When the child cries or strains the varix becomes engorged with blood.

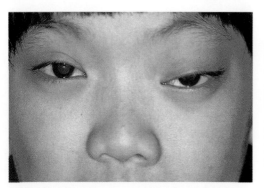
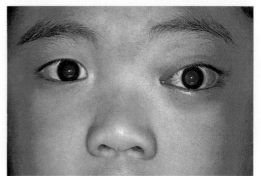

Orbital rhabdomyosarcoma causing forward and downward displacement of the left eye.

Forward displacement of the left eye due to neuroblastoma spread from adrenal gland.

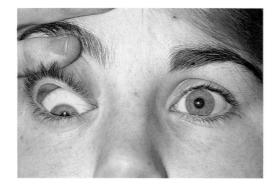

Orbital pseudotumour is a chronic inflammatory mass. When the lid is lifted the eye is displaced inferiorly by the lesion.

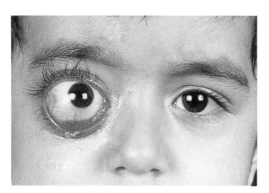

Proptosis of right eye in a child with neurofibromatosis.

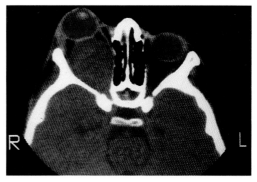

CT Scan shows mass behind right eye which proved to be glioma.

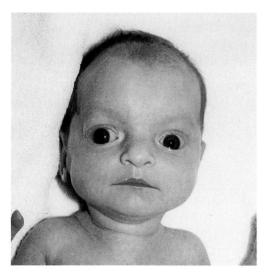

Infant with shallow orbits at risk of corneal exposure.

PART SEVEN

Systemic disease and the eye

Visual handicap

Systemic disease and the eye

Many chromosomal abnormalities, syndromes, and metabolic disturbances are associated with eye disorders. Recognition of the ocular manifestation often helps in the diagnosis of the systemic disease and optimal care for the child is only possible through the combined efforts of ophthalmologist, paediatrician, and general practitioner.

Albinism

Albinism is associated with impaired pigmentation which may be generalized or confined to the eye and is associated with photophobia, nystagmus, and reduced vision. The pigment contained in the choroid is deficient and macula development is poor. There is a lack of retinal pigment and neural miswiring at the chiasma and lateral geniculate body causing faulty binocular vision. In later childhood, special occluder contact lenses or tinted glasses may relieve troublesome photophobia.

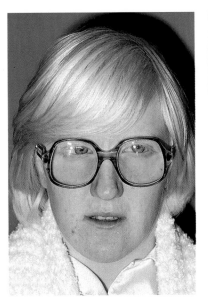

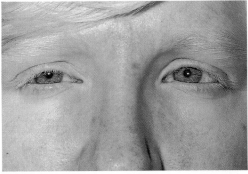

White hair and lashes of a tyrosinase-negative albino.

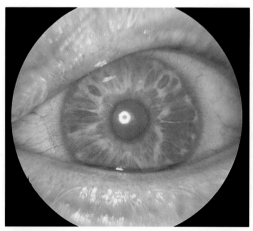

Albinism: the iris appears pink because of absent pigment.

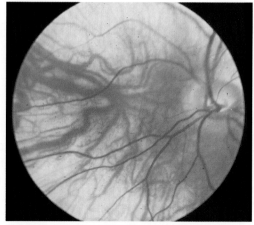

The retina appears pale with prominence of the retinal and choroidal vessels against the white of the sclera.

Aniridia

In this familial condition there is absence of the iris apart from a peripheral frill. Poor vision, photophobia, and nystagmus are present. Photochromic spectacles or dark goggles help to relieve photophobia. Cataract, glaucoma, and peripheral corneal scarring may develop in later childhood. There is an association between sporadic aniridia and Wilm's tumour.

Aniridia. Courtesy of Dr Alistair Blair.

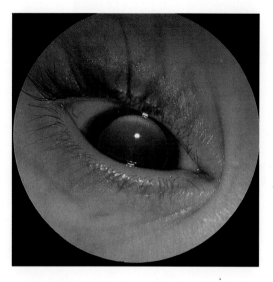

Down's syndrome

Down's syndrome or trisomy 21 is associated with chronic blepharitis, refractive error, squint, conical cornea or keratoconus and cataract.

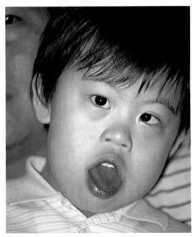

Down's syndrome. The child has a left convergent squint.

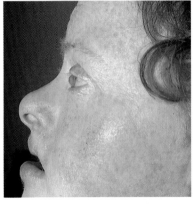

Down's syndrome. The corneal contour bulges forward abnormally, a sign of keratoconus.

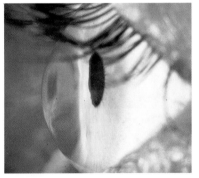

Keratoconus with obvious corneal bulging.

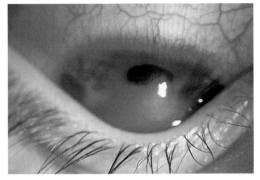

Keratoconus has led to corneal oedema at the apex of the cone which indents the lower lid on downgaze (Munson's sign).

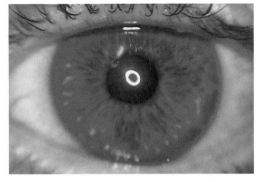

Down's syndrome. Brushfield spots on the iris.

Marfan's syndrome

Marfan's syndrome is a dominantly inherited condition associated with lens subluxation and dislocation, cataract, high myopia, and retinal detachment. The skeletal features of arachnodactyly (long, thin spindly fingers and toes), hyperextensible joints, kyphosis, high arched palate, and osteoporosis are typical.

Homocystinuria is a recessively inherited condition also associated with lens dislocation and skeletal changes similar to Marfan's syndrome are seen.

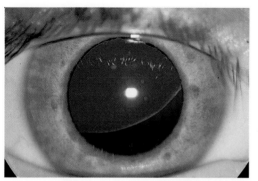

Marfan's syndrome. The edge of the subluxed lens is seen.

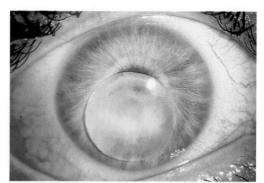

Homocystinuria. The cataractous lens has dislocated into the anterior chamber. Glaucoma will result unless the lens is removed.

Phakomatoses

The phakomatoses are a group of disorders with eye manifestations. They are usually familial or hereditary diseases giving rise to multisystem congenital hamartomas of neuroectodermal tissue. Four examples are neurofibromatosis or von Recklinghausen's disease, tuberous sclerosis, angiomatosis retinae or von Hippel Lindau disease, and cephalofacial angiomatosis or Sturge–Weber syndrome. Glaucoma can result from involvement of the anterior filtration angle with nodular tumours (von Recklinghausen's) or vascular malformations may impede the absorption of aqueous fluid (Sturge–Weber). Retinal angiomas can leak and impair vision (von Hippel–Lindau) or isolated fibrous hamartomas (tuberous sclerosis) may be found.

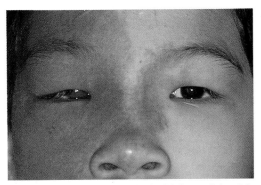

Sturge–Weber syndrome. The bluish haze of the right cornea indicates oedema due to glaucoma.

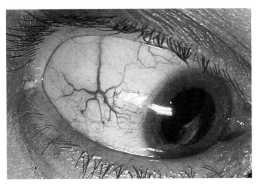

Abnormal blood vessels beneath the conjunctiva associated with Sturge-Weber syndrome.

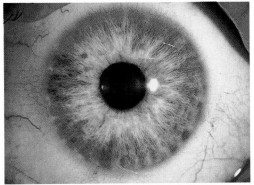

Neurofibromatosis. Lisch nodules on the iris. The child presented with proptosis and visual loss due to optic nerve glioma.

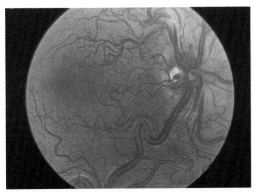

Von Hippel–Lindau syndrome. Retinal angiomatosis leads to dilated tortuous vessels. The child also has cerebellar haemangiomablastoma.

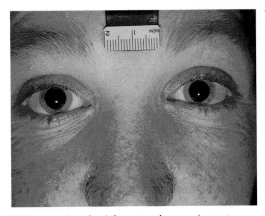

Tuberous sclerosis. Adenoma sebaceum is most commonly seen after two years of age.

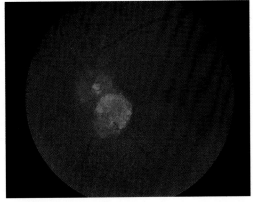

Tuberous sclerosis. 'Mulberry tumour' in the retina of a child with seizures and mental retardation.

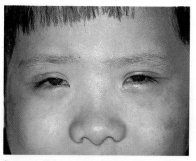

Stevens–Johnson syndrome. The child has photophobia due to corneal involvement.

Retinitis pigmentosa

This may occur in isolation or be part of a syndrome—Lawrence–Moon–Biedl syndrome, Usher's syndrome or Refsum's syndrome (see Part 3).

Stevens–Johnson syndrome

Stevens–Johnson syndrome is a hypersensitivity reaction usually to sulphonamide derivatives or infection causing conjunctival ulceration and scarring; this may lead to a dry eye, corneal ulceration, and severe visual disability. Ophthalmic referral is advised.

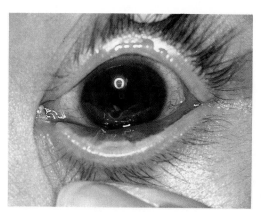

Stevens–Johnson syndrome. Abnormal deposition of keratin looks opaque in the lower tarsal conjunctiva.

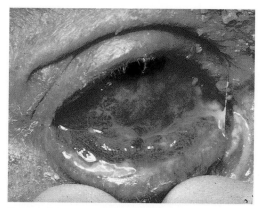

Stevens–Johnson syndrome. Severe conjunctival ulceration and repeated secondary infection leads to scarring and trichiasis. Blindness may result from corneal ulceration and infection.

Juvenile chronic rheumatoid arthritis (JCA)

JCA is associated with inflammation in the anterior chamber (iritis). Girls with pauciarticular JCA are at particular risk and both eyes may become affected. A child with JCA and iritis has a white and painless eye, unlike the adult with iritis. Iris/lens adhesions or posterior synechiae result in a distorted poorly reactive pupil. Treatment includes mydriatics and steroids. If left untreated, cataract and glaucoma may develop, therefore regular ophthalmological reviews are recommended.

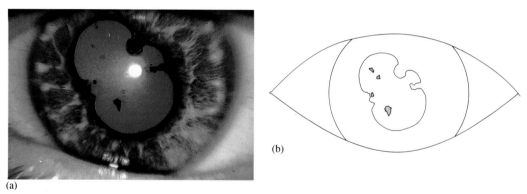

(a)

(b)

(a) Juvenile chronic rheumatoid arthritis associated with uveitis and posterior synechiae formation. The pupil is irregular and points of iris/lens adhesion are revealed after dilation. (b) The hatched areas are islands of pigment from the iris adherent to the anterior capsule of the lens. The pupil is irregular due to the firm adhesions between iris and lens at the one, two, and eight o'clock positions.

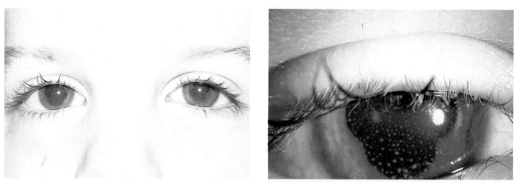

Treatment consists of mydriatics to prevent further posterior synechiae, and steroid to reduce ocular inflammation. Keratic precipitates can be seen as spots on the corneal endothelium and are clumps of cellular debris.

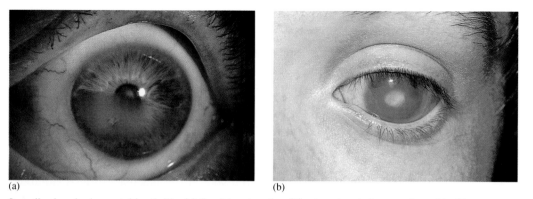

(a)

(b)

Juvenile chronic rheumatoid arthritis. (a) Band keratopathy, (b) cataract and glaucoma in a girl with pauciarticular rheumatoid disease.

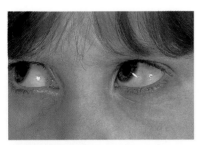

Osteogenesis imperfecta. Blue sclera associated with brittle bones and conductive deafness.

Osteogenesis imperfecta

Osteogenesis imperfecta or brittle-bone disease shows eye changes including thin sclera which appears blue, like fine porcelain, due to the enhanced visibility of the choroid.

Ehlers–Danlos syndrome

This is associated with angioid streaks, which are lines mimicking retinal blood vessels, but are really splits deep in the retina. Other ocular features include blue sclera, subluxated lens, and keratoconus.

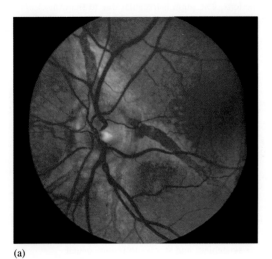

(a)

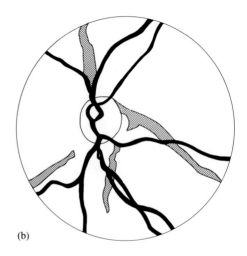

(b)

(a) Ehlers–Danlos syndrome. Angioid streaks are 'cracks' deep in to the retina (shown as hatched areas in line diagram), beneath the retinal blood vessels (solid lines).

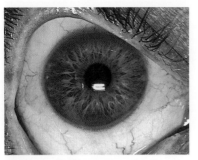

Wilson's disease. A brown peripheral corneal stain—a Kayser–Fleischer ring is associated with basal ganglia degeneration and cirrhosis.

Wilson's disease

Wilson's disease is a disorder of copper metabolism and may be accompanied by a granular deposit, believed to contain copper, in a ring at the edge of the cornea.

Neurometabolic disease

Neuronal storage diseases are associated with the degeneration of neurones in the retina and the appearance of a cherry red spot at the macula. Corneal clouding, glaucoma, retinal degeneration, and optic atrophy are ocular features of the mucopolysaccharidoses.

Ataxia-telangiectasia

This is associated with telangiectasis of the exposed conjunctival surfaces and nystagmus.

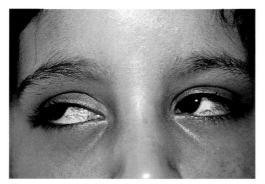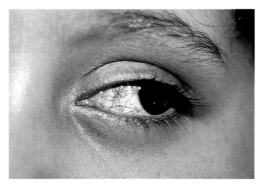

Ataxia telangiectasia or Louis–Bar syndrome. Telangiectatic and tortuous vessels in bulbar conjunctiva in a child with progressive cerebellar ataxia.

Visual handicap

Sight is the primary coordinating sense through which the child can relate to and explore the outside world. Vision allows information collected through the other senses to be given a definite meaning, without which, perception of the surroundings becomes a confusing jumble of noises, smells and tastes.

A blind child is unable to establish an early form of mother/child bonding through eye-to-eye contact. Other subtle forms of non-verbal communication are delayed such as facial mobility and pointing to surrounding objects of interest and frustration at this inability to make himself understood can lead to isolation and withdrawal into a trance-like state. Such a child will poke his fingers vigorously into his eyes in an attempt to evoke some form of visual stimulation. The development of a blind child is delayed particularly with head lifting, grasping, and crawling. Walking is not as delayed, and physiotherapy enhances progress with mobility.

The blind child has to be helped to reconstruct an impression of the environment using sound, particularly verbal communication, and touch. Smells and taste assume especial importance. Sudden noises can startle and softly spoken tones are to be encouraged. Once the child has enough confidence in himself and his surroundings, exploration will begin and this should be encouraged.

On hearing the news that their child is visually handicapped the parents react with shock, denial, and often anger. Some parents may lose the ability to cope with looking after a visually handicapped child not least because repeated hospital visits impose a strain in addition to the overwhelming emotional stress. It is only by sympathetic and honest explanation of the eye problem and patient counselling that the parents will come to accept and adapt to the situation. The social worker and home teacher for the blind are able to work with the family and support, advise, and mobilize welfare resources while the child is resident at home. Community self-help groups fulfil the function of allowing the parents of visually handicapped children to meet and discuss common difficulties and provide mutual support. There exists a range of visual disability from partially sighted to an inability to perceive even a light. Between these extremes are 'counting fingers' and 'hand movement' vision which may just allow a child to navigate safely and greatly reduces his degree of dependence. Many countries have a register which identifies and documents children with visual handicap and permits the welfare services to monitor and support both parents and children. In the UK about 500 children per year are registered as blind or partially sighted.

Mainstream schooling is preferable, providing the child has sufficient visual function and individual support to learn in this environment. Reading vision determines whether the child is placed in a school which has special educational equipment such as magnifying devices to aid close work and Braille books. Magnifying devices are available to make full use of a limited visual potential and include simple magnifying glasses or more expensive closed circuit television. A child with profound visual disability often has other handicaps such as cerebral palsy or deafness. Additional physical or mental handicap is present in up to 80 per cent of children on the blind register. Visual disability should always be considered when assessing the multi-handicapped child and early ophthalmic referral allows treatment of conditions such as cataract and glaucoma. The multi-handicapped blind child requires help from speech therapists, physiotherapists, and specially trained teachers; he may be better placed in a school which caters for such disabilities.

Preventing visual handicap

Preventable causes of visual handicap in children include:

Vitamin A deficiency

On a worldwide scale, vitamin A deficiency is the leading cause of preventable blindness afflicting the malnourished children of developing countries. Early

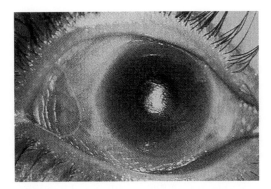

Vitamin A deficiency. Dry eye. Desiccated folds of conjunctiva with lacklustre cornea.

detection and treatment is important to save sight and save lives. Night blindness, conjunctival and corneal drying is followed by necrosis and perforation of the cornea. These progress rapidly and without signs of inflammation. Massive doses of oral and intramuscular vitamin A should be given immediately and supplements continued on a long-term basis. Prevention through community surveillance is important in areas with poor nutrition to identify those children at risk, and provide nutritional food, vitamin supplements, and dietary advice to families.

Trachoma

Trachoma is caused by *Chlamydia trachomatis* and is of a different serotype to the organism which causes sexually transmitted chlamydial eye infection. Trachoma is endemic in many parts of the developing world and is a cause of blindness in later adult life. The organism is spread by flies, fingers, and contaminated linen producing a recurrent infection mainly affecting the conjunctiva hidden beneath the upper lid. This leads to subsequent scarring in later life, pulling the eyelash-bearing upper lid margin inwards which abrades the corneal surface and predisposes to subsequent ulceration. Subnutrition encourages secondary bacterial corneal infection and indolent ulceration.

Treatment is to encourage hygiene and in particular face washing with clean water, which remains a luxury in many parts of the world. Topical tetracycline ointment is regularly applied three times a day for two weeks each month for six months, with regular community surveillance for signs of recurrent infection.

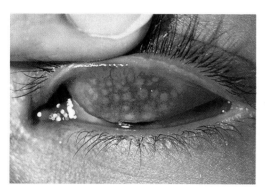

Trachoma. Upper tarsal conjunctival follicles in the early stages of the disease.

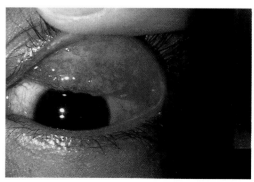

Later in life subconjunctival scarring causes trichiasis and its blinding sequelae.

Ophthalmia neonatorum

In many parts of the world where perinatal services remain poor, gonococcal ophthalmia is a preventable cause of misery and visual handicap. Prophylaxis using topical silver nitrate is effective though it can cause a chemical conjunctivitis; topical erythromycin is preferable if available.

Trauma prevention

Eye injuries are physically and emotionally traumatic for child and parent. It is especially tragic if the other eye is amblyopic or if both eyes are injured. Prevention involves giving advice to parents regarding potentially dangerous toys, and putting sharp objects well out of reach. In many parts of the world children have access to weapons including firearms, posing a threat to vision and life.

Genetic counselling

Eye abnormalities associated with a genetic cause are a leading cause of childhood visual handicap in the West. A combined approach from the ophthalmologist and geneticist working with the parents offers a method of primary prevention of visual handicap.

Antenatal diagnosis by the identification of the genes responsible for eye disease, such as X-linked retinitis pigmentosa and retinoblastoma, will soon be available.

Although the mother can be offered abortion of a fetus with such a defect, this may be refused, therefore, it is uncertain how effective this method of preventing visual handicap will be.

Formulary

Multi-application bottles containing eyedrops with preservative are available for individual use and may be used for up to one month. Single dose minims contain no preservative and should not be used more than once. Mydriatics, fluorescein, and local anaesthetic are available in minim-form, for use in the surgery or outpatient clinic. Most eye medications are available in ointment form for more prolonged drug action overnight.

Topically applied medication enters the eye by absorption through the cornea. It is also absorbed by the moist and vascular mucosal surfaces of the conjunctiva, and after passage down the nasolacrimal duct, by the nasopharynx. Side-effects may result from the systemic absorption of eye medications, such as cardiovascular effects of phenylephrine drops used to dilate the pupil, or the respiratory complications of topical β-blockers used in the treatment of glaucoma.

Administration of eyedrops into the eye of a reluctant child may be difficult—the likelihood of effective instillation is minimized by forcible lid closure and tears of distress dilute and wash away the medication. One effective method of applying eyedrops is to lay the child supine, and place the drop on to the inner aspect of the closed lids which are then opened allowing entry into the eyes.

If two or more varieties of eye medications are prescribed, an interval of 10 minutes between instillations is necessary to prevent flooding of the fornices and overspill of the drops, and to limit the dilution effects of the different drugs.

Hydrophilic soft lenses absorb the preservative in eye medications and fluorescein can cause permanent staining, therefore contact lenses should be removed before dyes are applied and while topical treatment is being used.

Antibacterials

Excessive tearing which accompanies acute conjunctivitis leads to dilution and rapid elimination of the antibiotic; therefore frequent instillation 2 hourly is required for the first few days till a response is observed, after which the frequency is reduced to 6 hourly for a further 3–4 days.

Chloramphenicol 0.5% drops and 1% ointment has broad spectrum activity. There are reports of aplastic anaemia.

Framycetin sulphate (Soframycin) 0.5% drops and 0.5% ointment also has broad spectrum activity.
   Fusidic acid (Fucithalmic) 1% in gel base (liquifies on contact with the eye) is effective in treating staphylococcal infection and is applied twice daily.

Tetracycline hydrochloride ointment is used in the treatment of trachoma infection.

Antivirals

Acyclovir (Zovirax) 3% ointment applied five times daily and for 3 days after healing for herpes simplex corneal infection.

Vidarabine (Vira-A) 3% ointment applied five times daily for herpes simplex corneal infection.

Anti-inflammatories

Corticosteroids should not be used for undiagnosed red eye conditions as dendritic ulcers are aggravated, and steroid glaucoma and cataract are associated with their use. For the same reasons combination drops of antibiotic/steroid preparations should be avoided unless the child is under the close supervision of an eye specialist.

Fluoromethalone 0.1% (FML) is a relatively weak steroid with a reduced tendency to cause steroid glaucoma

Prednisolone sodium phosphate (Predsol) 0.5% is an intermediate strength steroid

Prednisolone acetate (Pred-Forte) 1% and betamethasone sodium phosphate (Betnesol) 0.1% are relatively potent steroids

Non-steroidal anti-inflammatory drugs include sodium cromoglycate (Opticrom) 0.2% drops four times daily or 4% ointment 2–3 times daily, and lodoxamide (Alomide) 0.1% drops four times daily (children over 4 years). Vernal disease and other allergic forms of conjunctivitis may be treated with these preparations.

Mydriatics and cycloplegics

Both dilate the pupil and in addition cycloplegics paralyse the ciliary muscle responsible for accommodation, which renders the child unable to focus near objects.

To facilitate ophthalmoscopy tropicamide (Mydriacyl) 0.5% drops are an effective mydriatic with weak cycloplegic action; they act within 20 minutes and their action has a duration of 3 hours. In order to dilate the pupil and prevent posterior synechiae formation in the treatment of uveitis, phenylephrine hydrochloride 2.5% (Neo-synephrine) is combined with a cycloplegic agent.

For examination of refraction in young children, atropine sulphate 0.5% or 1% ointment is applied to each eye twice a day 1 or 2 days before the examination, and to treat uveitis atropine 0.25–2% drops are used in combination with phenylephrine drops several times a day. Atropine is a long acting cycloplegic with a duration of action in excess of one week. Contact dermatitis may occur, and toxic reactions resulting from systemic absorption can produce symptoms of flushing, fever, and restlessness.

Local anaesthetic

Proparacaine hydrochloride (Ophthaine) 0.5% drops is the least irritating of the topical anaesthetics, acting within 20 seconds and has a duration of action of 10–15 minutes.

Diagnostic dye

Fluorescein sodium 2% drops or sterile paper strips (wetted before use) are used to detect corneal ulceration and injury.

Further reading

Isenberg, S. (1989). *The eye in infancy*. Year Book Medical Publishers Inc.

Taylor, D. S. I. (1990). *Paediatric ophthalmology*. Blackwell Scientific Publications, Oxford.

Index